P9-DIG-238

Epilepsy
A New Approach

DATE DUE

DEMCO, INC. 38-2931

RC
372
.R53
1995

EPILEPSY

A New Approach

Adrienne Richard

AND

Joel Reiter, M.D.

Foreword by Robert Efron, M.D.

Walker and Company
New York

KVCC KALAMAZOO VALLEY
COMMUNITY COLLEGE
LIBRARY

Copyright © 1990, 1995 by Adrienne Richard

The ideas, procedures, and suggestions contained in this book are not intended to replace the services of a trained health professional. All matters regarding your health require medical supervision. You should consult your physician before adopting the procedures in this book. Any applications of the treatments set forth in this book are at the reader's discretion.

The cases and examples cited in this book are based on actual situations and real people. Names and identifying details have been changed to protect their privacy.

All rights reserved. No part of this book may be reproduced or transmitted in any form or by any means, electronic or mechanical, including photocopying, recording, or by any information storage and retrieval system, without permission in writing from the Publisher.

Originally published in hardcover in the United States of America in 1990 by Prentice Hall Press; this revised, paperback edition published in 1995 by Walker Publishing Company, Inc.

Published simultaneously in Canada by Thomas Allen & Son Canada, Limited, Markham, Ontario

Some of the material in this book has appeared in slightly different form in the magazine *Medical Self-Care* (May/June 1988), under the title "Self-Help for Seizures"; in the journal *Psychological Perspectives* (Fall 1987), as "The Fiery Wheel: Images and Experiences of Epilepsy"; and in the bulletin *Einfälle* (Number 18 and Number 19, 1986), published in West Berlin.

All illustrations are adapted from *Taking Control of Your Epilepsy: A Workbook for Patients and Professionals*, by J. Reiter, D. Andrews, and C. Janis, The Basics, Santa Rosa: California, 1987, with kind permission from the Andrews-Reiter Epilepsy Project, Inc.

Library of Congress Cataloging-in-Publication Data
Richard, Adrienne.
    Epilepsy : a new approach / Adrienne Richard and Joel Reiter ;
foreword by Robert Efron.
      p. cm.
    Originally published in hardcover : New York : Prentice Hall,
1990.
    Includes bibliographical references and index.
    ISBN 0-8027-7465-2
    1. Epilepsy—Popular works. I. Reiter, Joel. II. Title.
RC372.R53 1995
616.8'53—dc20   95-3651
                                   CIP

Original book design by Stanley S. Drate/Folio Graphics Co. Inc.
Illustrations by Ellen Gleeson

Printed in the United States of America

10 9 8 7 6 5 4 3 2

For Jim, 1916–1992, who stayed by me
through everything.

—AR

For Eleanor (Parady) O'Reilly.

—JMR

CONTENTS

ACKNOWLEDGMENTS

In the course of researching and writing this book, and in thinking about epilepsy in its many facets and contexts, I have been stimulated, challenged, and helped by many people in the United States and elsewhere. My debts are so numerous that I cannot acknowledge them all. I have been particularly encouraged along the way by my husband, Jim, and my three sons, Jim, Dan, and Randy. In the medical profession, Eugene Smith helped me to strengthen the initial insights and enlarge my vision. After every visit, Simeon Locke, chief of neurology at the New England Deaconess Hospital, Boston, sent me in new directions with his challenging questions and statements. Ulrich Hutschenreuter, neurologist and psychiatrist in Saarbrücken, West Germany, and a beloved friend, gave me the first validation that this material was publishable when he translated an early abbreviated version for a German publication.

I am especially indebted to the people around the country who called and wrote to tell me about sources of information, books, and articles that I might have otherwise missed. Louise Mahdi, Edith Sullwold, and Rosella Howe particularly come to mind. Often one person led to another who led to another. For instance, Edith Sullwold called to tell me of Lyall Watson's book *Lightning Bird*, and my correspondence with Dr. Watson in London led to sources in South Africa, where the medical librarian of the University of Witwatersrand dug out further rich and rewarding material. Another such source was Mary Gilbert, Ph.D., of the federal Environmental Protection Agency's Health Effects Research Laboratory in North Carolina. Our telephone conversation about seizures led her to send me research reports on the effects of caffeine on seizures that I had not seen before. Many such serendipitous trails led me into areas I had not yet explored.

My personal experiences in working with people with seizures were the most rewarding of all. At first I counseled only a few individuals. Then Meredith Sabins, R.N., gave me the opportunity to work with individuals with seizures at the James L. Maher Rehabilitation Center in Middletown, Rhode Island, where I discovered that the methods I had read about in the medical and psychological literature really did work. This discovery was validated further in the Boston-area workshops for persons with seizures that I have led with neurologist Harold Schiff. The contributions to this book made by the participants in those workshops are beyond measure. I cannot conceive of the book without them. The experiences of Jim, Tom, Carol, and the indomitable Marilyn spring immediately to mind. Each individual's story struck me as having a precious and sacred quality.

In the course of researching the vast material on epilepsy I was immeasurably assisted by a number of great libraries and their indefatigable reference librarians who thrive on tough questions. I made repeated use of the incomparable collection at the Countway Medical Library of Harvard Medical School, and I sat for many hours in the great vaulted reading room of the Boston Public Library, perusing nineteenth- and twentieth-century literature on epilepsy. The computerized National Epilepsy Library at the Epilepsy Foundation of America in Landover, Maryland, and its librarians, especially Robyn Ertwine, never failed to bring answers to my questions.

The literary agent Mildred Marmur steered this book to

its hardcover and softcover editions, and I am grateful for her experience, skill, and commitment.

The typing I did myself.

—ADRIENNE RICHARD
Stone Gate Vineyard
Westport, Massachusetts

Many people have contributed to my understanding of epilepsy, especially my patients, who will go unnamed but not forgotten. Donna Andrews is a continuing source of ideas and inspiration. I would like to thank Phyllis Grannis and the board of the Andrews-Reiter Epilepsy Project, Inc., for allowing us to use material from *Taking Control of Your Epilepsy: A Workbook for Patients and Professionals.* Dr. Michael Samuels has provided a unique perspective into self-care issues and medical philosophy through many years of dialogue. I am grateful to Dr. Sheldon Losin for covering my practice and encouraging my work. Dr. Irving Janis has given me valuable up-to-date references in behavioral medicine. Dr. Robert Hamburger assisted me by arranging a crucial interview. Most important, my wife, Charlotte Janis, has helped me immeasurably through stimulating conversation, excellent editing, and love.

—JOEL M. REITER, M.D.
Santa Rosa, California

FOREWORD

The basic thesis of this book is that many individuals with epilepsy can reduce the frequency of their seizures, and in some instances eliminate them entirely, by using a variety of techniques in addition to the anticonvulsant medication(s) that their physicians have prescribed.

A variety of safe techniques, some of which have been known for more than two thousand years, are well described. Despite the fact that medical science has not explained why these techniques are effective, there is no doubt that they do work for some people. Why then has the patient with epilepsy been so rarely told about them? There are two principal reasons.

The first is that many of these methods were developed when there was no other treatment for seizures. Once bromides were discovered to be useful at the end of the nineteenth century, and then even more effective anticonvulsant drugs became available in the twentieth century, chemical therapy for epilepsy became the medical treatment of choice. This tremendous medical advance quite understandably eclipsed these older techniques, of which few physicians today are even aware. Thus, even for those patients where chemical (and later neurosurgical) treatment is not fully successful in preventing seizures, the physician is usually unaware of these older techniques and, of course, never mentions them to his or her patients. For example, recently I gave a lecture at a leading university medical center in which I described how some of these archaic techniques are now being used again, at times with appreciable success. Not hiding his profound level of skepticism, the chairman of the neurology department asked at the end of my lecture whether any "reputable" neurologist (other than the invited speaker, of course) had ever used such methods for treating seizures. I quickly listed at least a dozen prominent neurologists, whose names he recognized instantly (including many who are quoted in this book), who had used these techniques successsfully and had described the results in the most respected medical journals. Several hours later, after he had done some library research, he ruefully acknowledged his ignorance of the history of treatment of epilepsy. Even this most distinguished academic neurologist was unaware that the techniques described in this book are often effective in reducing seizure frequency.

The second reason these techniques are rarely used today is that they require time-consuming experimentation by the patient as well as the physician. The patient must be prepared to make careful observations of all the circumstances surrounding each seizure (what he experienced before consciousness was lost, what other people who were nearby observed, etc.) and to document them in a notebook. With this information at hand, the patient and his physician (or counselor) can then experiment with the various techniques described here to see what can be accomplished on those occasions when anticonvulsant medication fails to provide complete seizure suppression, or when it produces medically undesirable side effects (during pregnancy, allergic reactions, etc.).

Joel Reiter, M.D., one of the coauthors of this text, is well aware of the potential value of these methods, and he uses them regularly. Furthermore, he works in conjunction with a trained epilepsy counselor to help his patients through the process of discovering the most suitable methods to improve seizure control.

Adrienne Richard, the principal author, heard about these procedures accidentally. Some years after she developed epilepsy she was referred to several of my articles published in Brain in 1956, 1957, and 1961, describing my work on the subject at a naval hospital. In the best tradition of the private detective, and with the help of the U.S. Navy Department, she managed to locate me more than twenty-five years after these publications. We had a long telephone conversation about how she might apply some of these techniques in her own case. I will not spoil her story by disclosing prematurely what she did next, except to say that she pursued the subject of seizure control with tremendous enthusiasm and determination. This research also led her to the more recently developed attempts to control seizures using biofeedback and meditation. This book not only describes her voyage of discovery but also contains a wealth of information about epilepsy not usually available to the general reader.

Among her discoveries is the fact that in more than 70 percent of individuals with epileptic seizures, there is some warning—an aura or other prodromal symptom—that gives the patient time to do something to abort the impending seizure. This book describes the many "somethings" that can be done if you have some warning that a seizure is about to occur. But even if you are among the 30 percent who have no warning at all, Adrienne Richard describes a number of other valuable things you can do to reduce seizure frequency.

The authors emphasize repeatedly that every individual with epileptic seizures is unique and that no single strategy—or even a medication—works for everyone. Thus, it takes a considerable amount of experimentation, time, and patience to discover which of these activities will work best for you. Although there is no guarantee of success, you have only your time to lose, and everything to gain!

—ROBERT EFRON, M.D.
School of Medicine
University of California, Davis
November 1989

PART ONE

THE EXPERIENCE OF EPILEPSY

═══════════════

[There is a] quest for a "new neurology," a holistic science of the person-with-the-illness, rather than the mechanistic and fragmented neurology of the illness itself.

—Samuel Shem

1

The Woman Who Sniffed Jasmine

. . . Each patient carries his own doctor inside him. They come to us not knowing that truth. We are at our best when we give the doctor who resides within each patient a chance to go to work.

—Albert Schweitzer, M.D.[1]

When I awoke with a piercing headache and began vomiting, my husband, Jim, told me that something had happened in the night. I had cried out, tossed about, and then lay still without waking up. Neither of us knew why or what had caused this strange occurrence, and since I was seven months pregnant, he wondered if he should leave me to go to work. I assured him that I would be all right, and he left.

All was well until mid-morning. My three-year-old son was playing near me on the living room rug when I felt a strange sensation beginning. I was stricken with panic. What was happening? What was I going to do? My husband was now thirty minutes away by car. We had recently moved to this midwestern city, and I didn't know my neighbors. If these sensations were a repetition of what had happened in the night, I did not want to go through that experience before the eyes of my little son who was completely dependent on me. The strange feelings increased. I picked up a toy or two and said, "Let's play in the bedroom. Mommy wants to take a little rest." My son followed me into the bedroom and settled onto the rug beside the bed.

3

I lay down, hoping he would see nothing, and stared hard at the ceiling. If I kept my eyes open, perhaps I could prevent this thing from overwhelming me. The strange sensations grew more powerful, and so did my terror. I stared hard at the ceiling, stared and stared, as the sensations increased. Then, to my astonishment, the feelings seemed to peak, stop, and then recede until they vanished. My heart slowed down, and I dared to blink my eyes. Exhausted, I propped myself on the pillows and spoke with my little son. He had noticed nothing.

The rest of the day went without incident. I was bewildered and tired, but there were no further episodes. That evening, however, with my husband at home and our son in bed, I was struck by another massive seizure. The next thing I knew it was morning and I was in a hospital bed. A strange doctor standing beside me was saying that he thought it was epilepsy.

Epilepsy? I stared at him in disbelief.

He wanted to do a few tests, he said, some x-rays of the head. A day later he was sure of his diagnosis. It was epilepsy. Again I stared at him. I had epilepsy? Epilepsy! A small voice inside me told me that I must never tell anyone. This disease was not socially acceptable. When my husband came to the hospital and learned of the diagnosis, we simply looked at each other, both of us agreeing without words that we must keep it a secret. Another, weaker voice also spoke, telling me that epilepsy was unusual, rather interesting, but it was silenced by the stronger voice of fear.

The doctor said he was going to put me on phenobarbital and Dilantin, two medications that should take care of the problem. Luckily for me and my unborn son, my pregnancy was into the third trimester and the fetus was not affected by these powerful drugs. It was not until three decades later that these drugs were recognized as potentially damaging to the fetus, especially in the first trimester.

From that time on, I took the medication compliantly, trusting that it would work, and it did. Several years passed. I then decided on my own that I no longer needed the drugs and dropped them. A massive seizure occurred a few months later, and I returned to the medication. I consulted eminent neurologists and went through diagnostic tests that became over time more sophisticated and more dependent on increasingly higher technology. I learned a little about my case—that the discharging lesion lay in the left temporal lobe of my brain and what the seizure spikes looked like on an electroencephalogram (EEG)—but the diagnosis never changed nor did the treatment.

When I was able to reflect on the initial diagnosis, I realized that the episode was not my first seizure but the first one to be observed by someone else. I had been aware of these feelings previously, but since they were minor episodes, I had not realized they were actually epileptic seizures. I had blamed these "feelings" on everything from fatigue to nerves. Now, thinking back over those early seizures, I am astonished to see their similarity. The seizure pattern over the years was always the same. They were all massive seizures with unconsciousness and some convulsion, the grand mal seizures that are synonymous with epilepsy. "Garden-variety epilepsy" one neurologist called it. In addition, I seem to have had the ability, when the seizures threatened during waking hours, to recognize the advance warning, the "aura" of fear and panic, even though I did not know such signals could occur. When I recognized the aura, I was able to exert control over the oncoming seizure. Nevertheless, it took me decades to learn that I could use this awareness of the aura systematically and consciously to stop a seizure from developing.

What astonishes me most now is that I immediately knew that I must never tell anyone about this affliction. If I did, I would be ostracized from normal social functioning. Although I was and am habitually curious and inquiring, I asked few questions, even of my neurologists. I sealed off my epilepsy in a secret compartment deep inside me. Only my husband, my parents, and my brothers knew. Epilepsy was a degrading thing to have.

How did I know this so instinctively at the instant of diagnosis? I had never thought about epilepsy before or been around it. Was it some buried residue from high school

English class where we read *Silas Marner*, the story of the linen weaver whose spells of epileptic unconsciousness brought false accusations and ostracism? I doubt it. I did not know then that the fear of epilepsy and the social stigma it continues to carry deeply affect everyone who has it. The very word seems to activate the most human of terrors, the fear of losing control, of losing the self, the shame of making a degrading public spectacle of yourself, the fear of death. It did not occur to me until years later that seeing epilepsy as "bad" was a perception, and one not held by all other cultures in the world, or even by all persons within our own culture. The medication controlled my seizures. For a long time I swallowed it and was silent.

I took anticonvulsants for two decades and had complete control over my epilepsy. Then, twenty years ago, I became aware of new approaches to health and healing, and I decided again to take the risk of going without medication. Over the course of a year or so I eased off the Dilantin and phenobarbital I had taken for twenty years. Abrupt cessation of anticonvulsants can precipitate seizures, but I didn't know this at the time. I was simply afraid to stop. At the same time my diet and life-style had changed. I learned yoga primarily to relax and strengthen my back fatigued by long hours at the typewriter. But in the process, I discovered the astonishing benefits in relaxation, in deep breathing, and in the practice of meditation. Osteopathic treatments helped me with the tension in my neck and shoulders. Over the past twenty years only two grand mal seizures have occurred. There have been some lesser episodes but nothing major. Eventually I began to wonder, what was I doing—or not doing—that accounted for this dramatic reduction in seizure activity?

One day I was talking with my neurologist about seizure reduction, and he said, "You know, you should read Robert Efron's work. You'll find it in the neurological journal *Brain* for 1957, maybe 1956." I went to the closest medical school library, found the journal, and under the unlikely title of "The Conditioned Inhibition of Uncinate Fits,"[2] I read a story about a woman who sniffed jasmine. Dr. Efron's patient was a concert singer whose seizures kept her from pursuing her career. Each seizure was preceded by a warning signal, an "aura," that manifested itself as the hallucination of a disagreeable smell. Dr. Efron gave his patient a small vial of essence of jasmine to sniff whenever she hallucinated this bad smell. It enabled her to stop her seizures before they went full course. Later he taught her through a process of conditioning how to imagine the odor of jasmine and stop her seizures by doing so.

When I read this account, I was astonished. Once again I looked at my own case and wondered. I remembered my experience of holding off a seizure as my three-year-old played on the rug beside me. In the opening paragraph of his article Dr. Efron noted: "Seizures spontaneously arrested during the aura are reported by almost every epileptic from time to time."[3] As I read this, years after that episode took place, my personal experience of epilepsy was validated for the first time. Had I unwittingly found a way to arrest a seizure? Did the diet and life-style changes I had now made constitute my own version of a sniff of jasmine?

Since then I have talked with many people who have epilepsy, and almost everyone has a similar story to tell of how he or she stopped a developing seizure. This curious experience of having some built-in control over a terrifying event—the sudden discharge of excessive electrical activity somewhere in the brain—opened my mind to new possibilities. Now I began to read more and more research studies that revealed we have much greater control over the unconscious processes of the body than we had formerly believed possible.

Soon after I read Dr. Efron's case study, I learned of the Mind/Body Workshops, an innovative program in self-care then being held at Beth Israel Hospital in Boston, and I wondered if the techniques taught there by Joan Borysenko and Steve Maurer would have an effect on seizures. I spoke with them, and in their next group I became part of an informal research project to investigate that very question.

There were two of us: a man of about thirty whose seizures began after a construction accident and myself. One of the techniques we learned during the ten weeks of the course was deep meditative breathing. Unknown to each other, we were both beset by seizures. When my colleague's massive grand mal seizure began with an aura of fear, he was able to use the deep breathing, dispel the fear, and stop the seizure from developing. My seizure or seizures involved a series of sensations of something taking me over like the ones I described at the opening of this book. This time, however, I was able to keep my body relaxed by closing my eyes, instead of staring hard at the ceiling, and breathing deeply. Just as they had years ago, the sensations peaked and receded. This time, however, I was able to dispel the fear. The episode was strange but pleasant, rather interesting, and not frightening at all.

After this experience, I was filled with great excitement. What else might reduce or control seizures? I had learned of biofeedback in the Mind/Body Workshop, and now I went to the Menninger Foundation in Topeka, Kansas, for training in its laboratory for the Voluntary Control of Internal Processes. There, under Elmer and Alyce Green[4] and Dale Walters, I learned methods of biofeedback that enabled me to control the temperature of my body, warming it at will. I learned how to relax my muscles and how to recognize the emotional effect of words, phrases, and tasks that increase or decrease the body's tensions. Particularly important for epilepsy were the brief experiments done with electrodes attached to my head to pick up the brain's electrical discharges. These showed me that even with a modicum of training the brain's electrical discharge could be altered voluntarily. I came home to investigate diet and found by reading the research that certain diets and certain nutrients helped to make the brain function normally. Of greatest interest to me were the many techniques available to arrest a seizure. Some were the simplest of behavioral methods. Others were like the smell of jasmine and involved sensory input, while still others depended on visualizations and complex mental images. I will describe all of these techniques later in this book.

What I have come to call my education through epilepsy led me into the long history of this disease/disorder and into the ways in which other cultures regard and treat it. It was illuminating to discover how our current biomedical view has appeared only recently. As medicine has changed, so has epilepsy. As historical and cultural contexts have shifted, epilepsy has been seen in a different light.

I searched through the anthropological literature and discovered that our western view of an epileptic seizure was not held by every society. Some cultures saw epileptic seizures as an evil, as the peoples of western Europe did a century and more ago, but others saw the seizures as the potential for great spiritual healing and divination. In those societies, people with epileptic seizures were not medically treated but trained for these great callings.

This cross-cultural and historical view opened my mind to a broader perspective on epilepsy than the one I had before. What's more, I discovered that there are neurologists within biomedicine, such as David Bear, M.D.,[5] who have taken into account the many historical personages who have had epilepsy or whose behavior suggests that they did. Would these people and their contributions in the realms of art, literature, religion, and politics be lost if epilepsy or the neurological conditions that underlie it did not exist? The question remains unanswered.

All of this material I found for myself by reading through the literature of neurology, psychology, medicine, and anthropology. Why had no neurologist ever mentioned any of it to me? I can only answer that question by citing Dr. Efron's introduction to this book. The education of the patient, and even more, the training of the patient in personal health care, has been neglected by modern medicine. The constraints of medical training, and a doctor's work load and fee schedule, limit what a physician is able to do and what a patient can afford.

Once my initial doubts were allayed, I grew more confident that the methods of self-care that I had stumbled upon could indeed be applied to seizures. Although I knew that they worked for me, I wondered if they would help others. The more I talked with people with epilepsy (I was really out in the open now) the more I realized that these methods would help many others as well.

My conviction was confirmed when I met a young neurologist in the Boston area who was also interested in a more broad-spectrum approach to epilepsy than simply the diagnosis and the treatment by anticonvulsants. With him and a psychiatrist, I began to give workshops for persons with seizures. The object of the workshops was to educate people about epilepsy and teach self-care skills and practices that would reduce the need for medication and help to control epileptic outbreaks.

The experience of teaching these workshops has been particularly gratifying to me. Almost everyone has been helped in some way. People learn about the neurology of epilepsy, information that had not been available to them previously. They learn and practice self-care methods that improve general good health and reduce exacerbating conditions. Most come to recognize the debilitating effects of stress and tension and the remarkably restorative powers of deep relaxed breathing.

When anyone reports the astonishing experience of blocking a seizure, it's always the highlight of that session. Particularly valuable, I believe, are the moments when someone says, "I can't believe I'm saying this to a group of people," or "I've never mentioned this to anybody but my doctor." Then I know that the secret compartment deep within has broken open.

I have followed a number of participants in these workshops over several years. They continue to use the techniques with success in reducing their seizures. You will hear from them throughout this book.

Primarily, however, I am a writer, and my research and experiences from the workshops began to take shape as journal and magazine articles. As I was preparing my article, "Self-Help for Seizures," for the magazine, *Medical Self-Care*, the editor, Michael Castleman, sent me a workbook put out by the Andrews/Reiter Epilepsy Research Program in Santa Rosa, California. To my amazement, I found many of the methods and techniques that I had come to on my own being used by a neurologist and an epilepsy counselor who worked with him. They, too, had found the new approach to epilepsy.

In the course of writing my article I talked with Dr. Joel Reiter on the telephone, and he expressed his concerns, long-standing since his days as a resident in neurology, about the toxicity of the medications used to treat epilepsy and the ineffectual treatment for some kinds of epilepsy. Since then we have met, become friends, and it is my pleasure to have Joel Reiter as collaborator on this book.

The years of study, research, and experience that have led to this book have been full of surprises and astonishments for me. Not the least of them is how one whiff of jasmine opened and altered my life. It awoke the "doctor inside" me, to use Dr. Schweitzer's words, broke the seal on the hidden compartment marked "unacceptable affliction," and stimulated my curiosity and inquiry in many new directions. One sniff and I set off on the healing journey that led to this book.

2

A New Approach
to Epilepsy

Healing is the process of wrestling with issues of meaning.
—Richard Katz, Ph.D.[1]

As medicine has moved more and more toward science, many aspects of the individual patient, his/her attitudes and values, life-style, feelings, dietary habits, and so on, are left out of the medical picture. Biomedicine, by and large, sees the patient as her symptoms, not as a whole person interacting with a diseased or disordered part.

Today this view has been challenged not only by so-called alternative healers and healing systems but by pioneers within biomedicine itself. Oliver Sacks, M.D., professor of neurology at Albert Einstein College of Medicine in New York and author of several books, is described by Samuel Shem as moving "forward in his quest for 'a new neurology,' a holistic science of the person-with-the-illness, rather than the mechanistic and fragmented neurology of the illness itself."[2] Psychiatrist and medical anthropologist Arthur Kleinman, M.D., has brought fresh insights to western medicine from his observations of traditional healers and shamans. They heal, Kleinman concludes, through their highly intuitive use of religious, emotional, and social support systems.[3] Research into the so-called placebo effect has shown the power of personal beliefs in the restoration of health. For some time now the effect of an individual's faith and hope on the course of some instances of cancer and heart disease has been widely reported. Herbert Benson,

M.D., the cardiologist who investigated the "relaxation response" and in whose department at New England Deaconess Hospital the Mind/Body Workshops flourish, has come to believe that a deep connection, revived if need be, with a religious tradition or spiritual life is an important component in a return to health.[4]

Although some doctors balk at changing their methods of patient care and others disparage the research that confirms the need to do it, the conviction is widely held that the more positive the patient's attitude and life-style, the greater hope there is for the outcome of an illness. Epilepsy is no exception. Even though it is long-term, often intractable, unpredictable, and idiosyncratic, it can be subjected to conscious control. There is a great deal that we who have seizures can do for ourselves, and we need to be involved in our own healing process.

Doing as much as we can to manage our own seizures has become more urgent in the past several years. The toxicity of the anticonvulsants used to control seizures is finally being addressed in public. A recent article in the *New England Journal of Medicine* begins, "Anticonvulsant drugs used to treat patients with epilepsy have long-term toxic effects. Therefore, prolonged treatment with these drugs should be avoided, particularly if satisfactory control of seizures has been achieved."[5] The medications that I took for two decades—phenobarbital and phenytoin (Dilantin)—are now recognized as causing chronic fatigue and depression. I battled both of these symptoms for years on end, not knowing that the medication I swallowed daily was perhaps causing and certainly exacerbating these conditions. Phenobarbital, the common drug for generalized seizures in children, affects cognitive development, even in small doses. Carbamazepine (Tegretol), which is given in large doses to many adults, is carcinogenic in laboratory rats. It is obviously important to keep dosages as low as possible over as short a term as possible, and self-care practices help to do this.

Current research on anticonvulsant medication confirms the option of short-term use. The study reported in the *New*

England Journal of Medicine suggests that adults with certain types of seizures who go seizure-free for a two-year period on medication will be highly likely to be seizure-free without medication thereafter. That the same is true for children has been confirmed by studies done at Johns Hopkins University under John G. Freeman, M.D.[6] The health-care practices delineated in later chapters of this book will reinforce and extend seizure-free periods.

In addition to the toxic effects on the body and negative effects on cognitive abilities such as memory, anticonvulsants affect other, more subtle, experiences. One neurologist has reported that his patient, a poet, told him that when the medication makes the seizures disappear, her poetic muse disappears as well.[7] A woman with a deep spiritual life told me that the religious experiences of her youth never occurred during the years of medication and since foregoing medication they have now returned, enriching her life. David Bear, M.D., the eminent neurologist with a persistent interest in the creative aspects of epilepsy, suggests that epilepsy may have a role in "transcendant artistic production." He cites Van Gogh, Dostoyevski, St. Paul, Moses, and Mohammed as persons whose life work may have been enhanced by epilepsy.[8] My Boston neurologist told me one day, "You know, I see a seizure as an aesthetic experience." Although few of us will be called to "transcendant" artistic or religious achievement, we do not want to lose unnecessarily such enriching and perhaps ennobling experiences.

Epilepsy, however, is not the sole property of the endowed and gifted. It afflicts persons at every level of intellectual functioning. In my work with retarded persons I have found that individuals with very restricted capabilities can learn self-care methods and even invent their own. In one research study a twenty-six-year-old man with an IQ of 49 learned the most sophisticated and difficult technique of biofeedback control of epileptic brain activity, reducing his seizures from nineteen a month to four.

In addition to the need to keep medications as low and as short-term as possible, epilepsy treatment is affected by the incomplete knowledge of the functions of the brain.

When a neurologist addressed a recent annual meeting of the Epilepsy Association of Massachusetts, he said, "We don't know everything." The audience responded with laughter and applause. As more is known, treatment will change. One particular area where knowledge is incomplete is in what Oliver Sacks, M.D., calls "the neurology of living experience,"[9] that is, the interconnections within the brain and between the brain and body that produce our individual thoughts and emotions, our imaginations and particular views of the world.

The essential characteristic of the new approach to epilepsy presented in this book is its comprehensiveness. It includes both medical care and self-care. Its emphasis is on our individual ability to think and care for ourselves. Our need to know and understand as much as possible about epilepsy underpins this emphasis. The outcome will be a greatly enhanced quality of life.

In Dr. Joel Reiter's West Coast practice of neurology all these aspects are included. If you had an appointment with him, he would listen to your history, perform a neurological examination, and order certain tests: an electroencephalogram (EEG) and a computerized tomography (CT) scan of the brain at a minimum. He would evaluate these tests and then prescribe the needed daily medication. In addition— and his practice exemplifies the new approach to epilepsy— you would have the opportunity to schedule a series of visits with an epilepsy counselor. In these counseling sessions you would learn what you needed to know to care for yourself better. You would learn how to recognize typical warning signals—the epileptic aura—and how to change exacerbating circumstances. You would learn what to do to improve your general and neurological health.

Joel Reiter's program is much the same program for self-care that I came to independently on the East Coast and taught in a group format. Such a program is hardly new in other areas of health care. In the treatment of heart disease such a comprehensive program involving the patient in his own healing process is not only commonplace but considered necessary. People with diabetes, for example, must understand their own case and learn what treatment they must follow. After my husband endured three days of hemorrhaging from the colon, the gastrointestinal specialist sat down with him and, using illustrations and x-rays, pointed out the problem areas, described gastrointestinal functioning, and prescribed the changes in diet and life-style my husband needed to make. As his principal supporter and cook, I was present, and his education became my education as well.

Epilepsy has not yielded to these newer medical practices. Why it hasn't, I believe, is a function partly of its history. We are willing to discuss our hearts, our tumors, and our colons with friends and acquaintances, picking up information and doctor referrals as we do so, but most of us are too afraid of and intimidated by epilepsy to speak or act openly. My diagnosis of epilepsy so frightened me that it prevented me for years from asking questions and getting the information I needed. I was too intimidated to bring my usual inquiring mind to this experience. This fear reinforces the long-held social taboos that surround epilepsy. It makes us more dependent than we need to be. In addition, the highly technical nature of neurological information makes it difficult for doctors to convey what we need to know. How the brain functions and what a seizure is and what it indicates are complex issues, and to a lay person, esoteric and bewildering as well.

Epilepsy, too, carries psychological, social, and legal complications that heart disease, diabetes, and even cancer do not. These complications and constraints often afflict the person with seizures more than the seizures themselves. Consequently, something more than the specialist's explanations with illustrations and x-rays is needed for the individual to learn how to live successfully with epilepsy.

This new approach to epilepsy has four principal aspects:

1. Your knowledge of epilepsy and its treatment
2. Your mental attitude
3. Your practice of a preventive program
4. Your ability to use methods of intervention.

Each one of these aspects will be addressed at length in the upcoming chapters, and each chapter will conclude with exercises and a suggested program for implementing that chapter's recommendations.

Your mental attitude toward your seizures begins with your decision to take control. The Santa Rosa team of Joel Reiter, M.D., Donna Andrews, Ph.D., and Charlotte Janis, F.N.P. write in their workbook, *Taking Control of Your Epilepsy*,[10] "Only your active participation in seizure control will enable you to reach your optimum level of wellness." Taking control is an active process predicated on your willing commitment to this decision.

This commitment is much easier for some people than for others. If you grew up as I did in a household where nontraditional health methods were practiced, it is likely to be easier. My mother dispensed homeopathic remedies when we were ill as children, using as her guide a booklet on homeopathy, the dominant form of medicine in the nineteenth century that was dying out as I grew up. In my mother's search for help with her terrible migraine headaches she drew on the health foods from Dr. Kellogg in Battle Creek, Michigan, the older brother of the cornflake king, so my after-school snacks were more likely to be vegetized crackers and malted nuts than Twinkies and Diet Pepsi. Consequently, my background makes it quite acceptable to me to find methods and remedies that are not mainstream biomedicine. In the area where I live a wholefoods supermarket chain has some of the most crowded stores in the region, making many chemical-free and wholegrain foods readily available, a far cry from the tiny healthfood stores my mother used to frequent. The new stores are a kind of socially acceptable nutritional support system for people who take self-care seriously.

The secrecy that surrounds epilepsy is another deterrent to taking control. It is difficult to embark on a program of self-care alone. Most people in my epilepsy workshops admit that they have never talked to anyone other than their immediate family and their doctors about their seizures. To build and maintain your attitude of taking control you need a supportive environment. In our self-care workshops participants become a support system for each other. Cheers go up when someone uses a method successfully, and the sense that "if he can do it, I can" is palpable in the group. Around the country there are many support groups for persons with epilepsy. Usually these are not self-care groups as well, but their importance as a forum to share experiences, to talk about alternatives, and to recognize the great variety of seizures that exist cannot be minimized.

Families should also be sources of strong support and help, but this is often not the case. The age old taboos surrounding epilepsy make acceptance difficult. In addition, persons with seizures can be very demanding, particularly if they are having difficulties in getting a job, problems on the job, or problems in their personal relationships, or if they have the types of seizures that carry nonrational behavioral components. All of us use our aches, pains, and illnesses to get that little extra bit of attention from the people around us, but anyone with a long-term problem needs to be aware that his demands may anger and irritate, even alienate, those he depends on most.

One consequence of the decision to take control is the giving up of the special status epilepsy may have given you. You may see yourself as a victim or as deserving of special privilege or special scorn. Once you take control, you can no longer say, "I'm an epileptic. I can't help it—I can't do it." Taking control means that you have decided to accept yourself as a person who has to deal with seizures as part—but not all—of your life.

Observing yourself is the key to both seizure prevention and intervention. Robert Efron, M.D., told me one day by telephone, "The critically important thing in epilepsy is observation of oneself both inside and out." Methods to observe carefully and minutely are contained in the chapter on observation. When self-observation breaks down, what is observed by another person can be almost as valuable. The interior events that precede a seizure, the seizure itself, and the circumstances that surround and put you at highest risk can be altered once they have been observed.

All the facets of preventing seizures are treated in detail

in Part Five of this book. Altering your circumstances; finding and building a supportive environment; releasing stress; breathing deeply; promoting relaxation and good nutrition; learning what substances improve brain function and what substances impair brain function; and identifying environmental hazards—all of these factors have been researched for their effects on seizures. Certain techniques seem to help persons with epilepsy more than others, and these are explained in detail with a suggested program for guidance.

Interventions are probably the most interesting and unusual aspect of this new approach. Some interventions are individual and internal, like telling yourself to be calm. Others are directly related to a characteristic in the aura such as fear or using the smell of jasmine to stop a seizure that begins with a smell. Others involve the amazing power of mental imagery. Still others are those interventions that can be employed by outsiders when they see you drifting into a seizure. How to discover your own interventions and how to use them systematically to arrest seizures is made clear in Part Six.

Again, understanding, information, mental attitude, observation, prevention, and intervention are the cornerstones of the new approach to epilepsy.

You are now embarking on a self-care program for seizures. Your commitment will help it work for you. Write the following on a piece of paper and put it on your refrigerator or bathroom mirror:

The brain is essential to life.
I want my brain to act calmly and normally.
I will do everything I can to help my brain act calmly and normally.

This book is designed and intended to be used by the reader. To use it well you will need a notebook: a three-ring binder where pages can be added, or a spiral notebook of at least eighty pages. At the end of each chapter there are instructions to be followed and questions to be answered, and your notebook is important for these purposes. Always leave space between entries—begin a new page for each one—so that you can return and enter additional notes. Don't concern yourself with spelling, punctuation, or sentence structure. These entries are for your use as you make your experiences of epilepsy more conscious and objective.

In your notebook, for your first entry:

- Describe your first seizure or the first one that you remember. Put down as much about it as you can—what the seizure was like, where you were, who was with you, what kind of seizure it was, what you did about it or what your family or those around you did about it, and how you felt afterward.
- Describe your feelings when you were first told that you had epilepsy. How do you feel now?
- Leave space to add to your personal account.

PART TWO

THE NEUROLOGY
OF EPILEPSY

Joel Reiter, M.D.

3

The Biomedical View of Epilepsy

Epilepsy is explainable as a dysfunction of some of the cells of the brain, which leads to dysrhythmia of action and paroxysmal seizures. With epilepsy as with most diseases (for example, diabetes, obesity, cancer, arthritis), the ultimate origin has been traced to the doorway of the cell, to intracellular mechanisms. We know more about the cause of epilepsy than about the cause of many diseases for which the complaint of "unknown" is seldom raised.

—Dr. William Lennox[1]

Adrienne Richard asked me to describe the brain events that result in seizures because I am a neurologist. When I think about epilepsy, some of my patients come to mind rather than the random electrical firing of nerve cells that results in their seizures. I became a doctor rather than a research neurophysiologist because as a doctor it is my job to correlate what my patients tell me about their experience of having seizures with the growing knowledge of medical science.

Physicians have described and ministered to people with epilepsy for millennia. In the fifth century B.C., Hippocrates placed epilepsy under the aegis of medicine when he said, "The disease called sacred is not in my opinion any more divine or more sacred than any other disease, but is of natural cause and its supposed divine origin is due to men's inexperience and to their wonder of its peculiar character."[2] The Greek physician Aretaeus, in the second century A.D., said, "In the attack, the person lies insensible; the hands are clasped together by the spasm; the legs not only plaited together, but also dashed about hither and thither by the tendons. The calamity bears a resemblance to slaughtered bulls; the neck bent, the head variously distorted."[3]

A little over a hundred years ago the great British neurologist John Hughlings Jackson ushered in a new era in the medical understanding of epilepsy. He attributed seizures to "an occasional, an excessive and a disorderly discharge of nerve tissue."[4] The medical challenge since Jackson's groundbreaking work has been to learn how nerve cells discharge, yet maintain a sense of order within the brain. For example, how can I focus my attention to type this chapter without my legs moving, my head turning, or my mind thinking of other things? In the act of writing, brain cells in my language center and in my motor strip discharge while brain cells in my talking speech area and in my leg area do not discharge.

Two different basic brain cell processes occur in my brain at the same time in order for me to write. Excitation occurs when one brain cell (neuron) tells another brain cell to fire electrically. Inhibition occurs when one neuron tells another neuron not to fire. If the processes of excitation and inhibition are balanced within my brain, I can function in my usual way.

A group of neurons within the brain will discharge excessively and randomly if too much excitation occurs or if too little inhibition occurs. If enough neurons discharge excessively at the same time a seizure will occur. When most of the neurons in the brain cortex discharge at the same time, a generalized tonic-clonic (grand mal) seizure occurs. Sometimes a small area of the brain contains neurons that tend to discharge excessively, but neurons in adjacent areas of the brain are able to prevent this excess discharge from spreading into their territory. Seizure activity remains confined to the brain area with excessive discharge. Neurologists call this occurrence a *partial seizure*. If the brain area with excessive discharge is very small, a person may experience an unusual sensation with no visible manifestation of a seizure. This sensation is called an *aura*.

The same person may experience an aura followed by a visible seizure if the excessive brain discharge spreads to involve a larger area of the brain.

In 1929, Dr. Hans Berger described a way to test for the excessive brain discharges that result in seizures. He discovered that the electrical activity of the human brain could be measured as a difference in electrical potential between two points on the surface of the scalp. He named this test the *electroencephalogram,* or *EEG.* Since he first described the EEG, it has become more sophisticated and easier to use. The painful pins used initially have been replaced by a set of twenty-two electrodes, which are pasted onto the scalp. Technicians connect these electrodes to an EEG machine, which produces pen and ink tracings of the brain's electrical activity.

As a neurologist, I can determine from an EEG pattern whether a person was awake, drowsing, asleep, or in between these states at the time the EEG was actually recorded. To read an EEG, I must know the range of normal as well as what is abnormal. People with epilepsy may have abnormal brain waves known as *spikes* or *sharp waves.* If a particular area of the brain has a tendency to develop excessive discharges, it may show intermittent spikes or sharp waves. In contrast, an abnormal brain area may be more quiet than normal between seizures; this pattern is called *slow wave activity.* Other people may have normal EEG patterns between seizures. With some patients, I can diagnose a particular type of epilepsy by looking at their EEGs. Others have normal EEGs and I must rely on their histories alone for diagnosis.

Recently my patients and I have been confronted with the new epilepsy classifications. A woman who has had grand mal seizures for years called me to ask if her seizures had changed. During a visit to her sister, she had a seizure and the neurologist she saw told her she had *generalized tonic-clonic seizures.* Another patient was taken aback when I told him he had *complex partial epilepsy.* He said that his neurologist in New York had diagnosed him with temporal lobe seizures years ago. *Absence* used to mean

Definitions:

Frequency = number of waves ("cycles") occuring each second, indicated as "cycles per second" (cps). cps is the same as the scientific term hertz (hz).

Amplitude = height of each wave, indicated in microvolts (μv).

Awake, active pattern:
Low amplitude 12–30 cycles per second (cps).
"Beta pattern."
Experienced as "alert, anxious, energetic, and/or tense."
Thinking, problem solving, worrying, decision making.
Seizures may occur in this state.

Awake, relaxed pattern:
Medium amplitude 8–12 cycles per second (cps).
"Alpha pattern."
Experienced as "passive, calm, unfocused, at ease."
May notice heightened body sensations, absence of thought.

Drowsy pattern:
Medium amplitude 5–7 cps.
"Theta pattern."
Experienced as "drifting, hazy, dreamy."
Seizures often take place during this state.

Sleep pattern:
High amplitude 1–4 cps.
"Delta pattern."
Experienced as sleep.

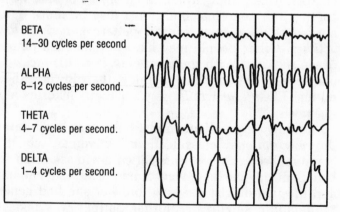

BETA
14–30 cycles per second

ALPHA
8–12 cycles per second.

THETA
4–7 cycles per second.

DELTA
1–4 cycles per second.

FIGURE 1.
Normal brain wave states as they appear on an EEG tracing.

"not present," but now it has replaced *petit mal*. For a while I tried to resist this changing terminology since it led to miscommunication with my patients. At this point, however, the new diagnostic classification system for epilepsy seems to be here to stay. Only the names for seizures have changed; the way seizures feel and look remains the same.

One hundred years ago British and French neurologists evolved a descriptive classification that was based on the visible appearance of seizures. Seizures with loss of consciousness and stiffening and/or jerking of the entire body were termed *grand mal*, which in French means "big badness." Seizures that involved altered consciousness without loss of consciousness were called *petit mal* for "little badness." When seizures involved only one part of the body they were called *focal*. More complicated seizures that featured both alteration of consciousness (psychic component) and involuntary movement of parts of the body (motor component) were termed *psychomotor* or *temporal lobe*.

Modern neurologists have devised a new classification that defines epilepsy according to whether the abnormal discharge arises from abnormal neurons on both sides of the brain (*generalized epilepsy*) or just part of the brain (*partial epilepsy*). Grand mal has been replaced by *tonic* if the body stiffens, *clonic* if the body jerks, or *tonic-clonic* if the body stiffens and jerks. Seizures that involve a lapse of consciousness caused by generalized brain discharge are termed *absence* rather than petit mal. All seizures that result from an abnormal discharge in an isolated area of the brain are termed *partial* seizures. Partial seizures without alteration of consciousness are termed *simple partial*. Partial seizures with alteration of consciousness are termed *complex partial* rather than temporal lobe or psychomotor.

In the remainder of this chapter, I will describe different types of epilepsy. I will associate the type of epilepsy with a description of the abnormal brain activity that causes it. I hope that by using the new descriptive classification of epilepsy, I will make it easier for you to talk with your neurologist.

TYPES OF EPILEPSY

GENERALIZED

Tonic-Clonic, Clonic, Tonic (Grand Mal). Before experiencing a generalized seizure, some of my patients know they are about to have a seizure. They report a vague feeling of unease, an odd feeling in the pit of their stomachs, or dizziness for a brief time before the seizure. Others have no warning at all. Many patients tell me they know when they have had a seizure by symptoms that follow afterward known as *postictal* symptoms. A small number tell me they wet themselves or bite their tongue during the seizure. More often symptoms of confusion, headache, or marked fatigue follow seizures.

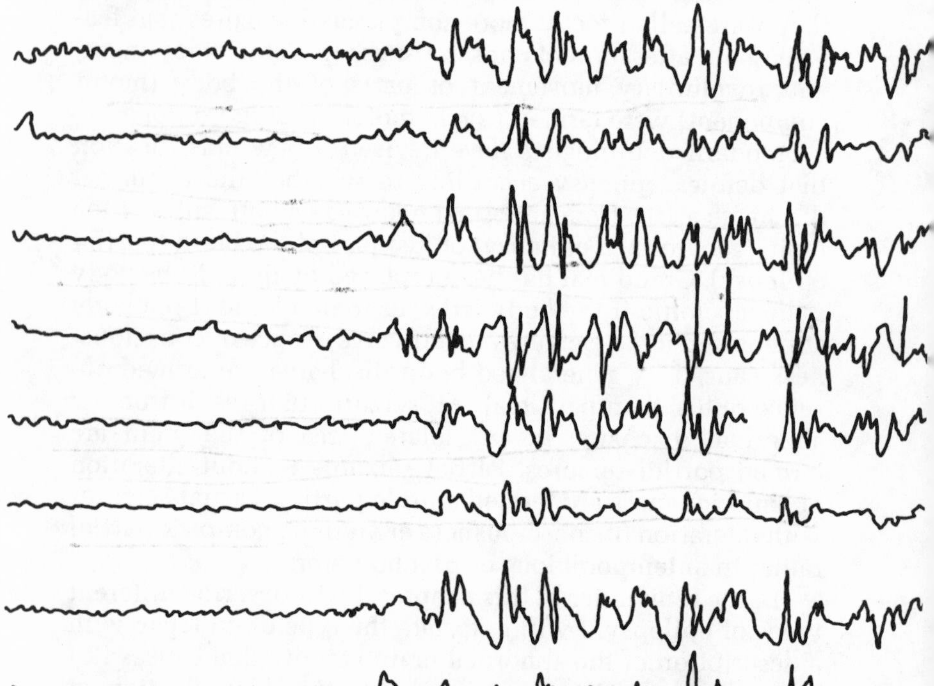

FIGURE 2.
Routine EEG shows a burst of polyspike activity in a patient who has intermittent generalized tonic-clonic seizures. Idiopathic epilepsy.

I don't witness my patients' seizures, so I rely on family members or friends to describe the seizures. Typically they describe passing out with stiffening of the entire body and clenching of the jaw (tonic phase). The observer reports that the patient looked blue and stopped breathing. Out of concern, some family members have tried to administer cardiopulmonary resuscitation (CPR). The blueness occurs because blood vessels in the skin constrict to allow more blood to go to the brain. In fact, blood flow to the brain increases fourfold to protect the brain during a seizure. After seconds to a few minutes, the stiffening of the body becomes random jerking of the limbs and torso (clonic phase) and then limpness.

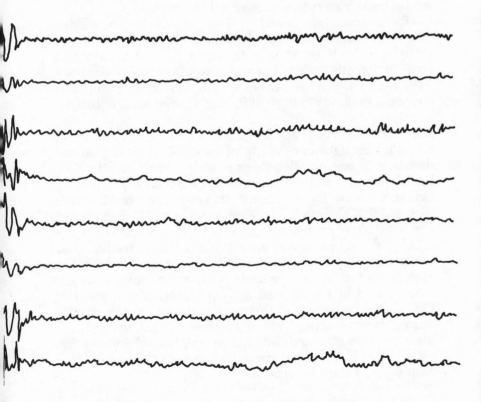

Many of my patients are more disturbed by what well-meaning onlookers try to do to protect them than by the seizure. Heather, who is now in college, remembers students trying to shove pencils into her mouth when she was having a seizure in high school. Her mother told me, "Kids said she was violent. They didn't know how to handle someone who's having a seizure. You should just move hard objects out of the way and leave them alone until it's over."

A twenty-eight-year-old man I saw recently asked me if there was truth in the writings of a French philosopher–poet he had read. The poet wrote that whenever he was about to reach nirvana, his being couldn't deal with the experience, so his mind and body separated, resulting in a seizure. I didn't know how to answer the question but replied that I am limited by an orthodox medical framework.

Tonic-clonic (grand mal) epilepsy results from a sudden discharge of most of the neurons in the brain. When all the brain cells discharge at once, the entire body stiffens. When some brain cells fatigue, but others continue to fire, the body jerks randomly. After all brain cells fatigue and stop discharging, the body is limp, the mind is tired and confused.

Absence Seizures (Petit Mal). When I was first in practice, a mother brought her delightful red-headed eight-year-old daughter to see me. Because the girl seemed so attentive, intelligent, and well behaved, it was hard for me to believe that she was having a difficult time at school. Her teachers reported that she made frequent mistakes on the blackboard and was often unable to answer simple questions. In my office, I asked her to take some rapid shallow breaths. After thirty seconds, she stared vacantly into space with her eyelids fluttering. Ten seconds later, she was back to her usual self. I had witnessed a classic absence seizure. Her EEG showed a pattern of three cps spike and dome activity during overbreathing, typical of absence epilepsy. After I placed her on ethosuximide (Zarontin), her schoolwork became exemplary. Now at age sixteen she has "outgrown" her epilepsy and is off medication.

School was even more problematic for Josh, a sixteen-year-old boy I saw two years ago. He was on the verge of getting expelled from a very good prep school because of inappropriate behavior. His teacher reported him for being on drugs because he would fade in and out of contact many times a day and then deny any problem. His father vacillated between being a strict disciplinarian and worrying. Josh appeared perfectly normal when I examined him. However, his EEG showed intermittent bursts of abnormal activity consistent with a diagnosis of juvenile absence epilepsy.

I wrote a letter to the teacher explaining my diagnosis. Since Josh had been burning the candle at both ends, his parents wanted to see if the problem would stop when their son got eight hours sleep every night and ate regular meals. Several weeks later, his mother was frantic because Josh's school had called to say that her son was confused and unable to communicate. His EEG showed continuous abnormal 3 cps polyspike wave activity, typical for a condition known as *absence status* in which the absence seizures become continuous. Now that his parents realized that Josh needed medication, he was started on Depakote, and he has had no problem with seizures for two years.

During an absence seizure, the part of the brain that keeps a person aware becomes disconnected from the brain cortex. The person loses contact, but not consciousness. Sometimes this loss of awareness is accompanied by a loss of motor function, which results in an abrupt jerk of body or limbs (myoclonic jerk), or in loss of muscle activity (akinetic fall). For some children absence seizures may be due to a lag in maturation of their brain chemistry, which could explain why many children "outgrow" absence epilepsy. Teenagers who experience absence seizures for the first time are diagnosed as having *juvenile absence epilepsy*. Juvenile absence epilepsy often requires medication into adulthood, and is

FIGURE 3 (overleaf).
Sixteen-year-old boy described in text who had continuous absence seizures at school. (a) During absence seizure; (b) After treatment

(a)

LEFT

LEFT

LEFT

LEFT

RIGHT

RIGHT

RIGHT

RIGHT

(b)

LEFT

LEFT

LEFT

LEFT

RIGHT

RIGHT

RIGHT

RIGHT

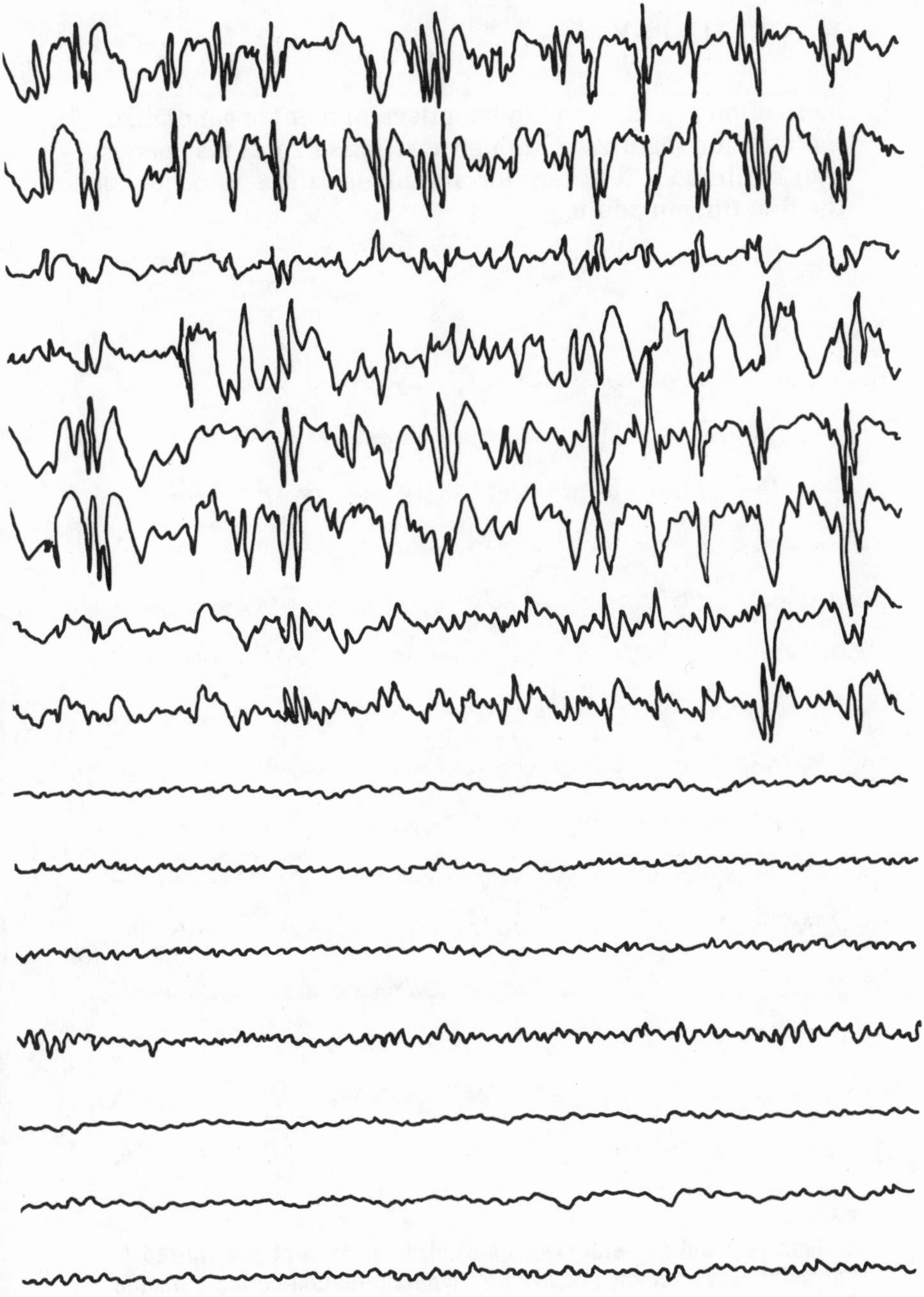

more often associated with later development of generalized tonic-clonic seizures. Although absence seizures may persist into adulthood, it is rare for absence seizures to occur for the first time in adults.

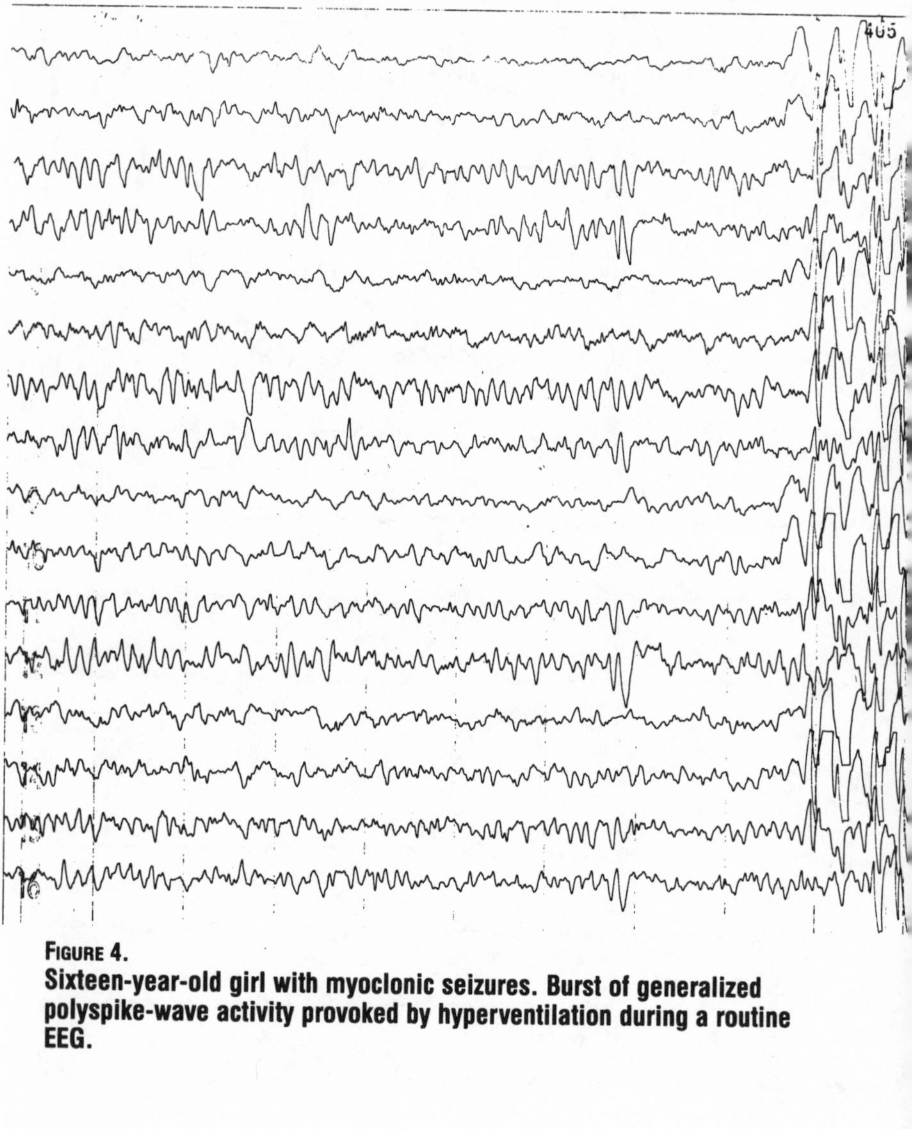

FIGURE 4.
Sixteen-year-old girl with myoclonic seizures. Burst of generalized polyspike-wave activity provoked by hyperventilation during a routine EEG.

Juvenile Myoclonic Epilepsy (Myoclonic Epilepsy). Seizures can first occur at inopportune times. A strapping farm boy came to see me after he had nearly fallen out of a hay truck. This industrious lad had gotten up at 4 A.M. to help

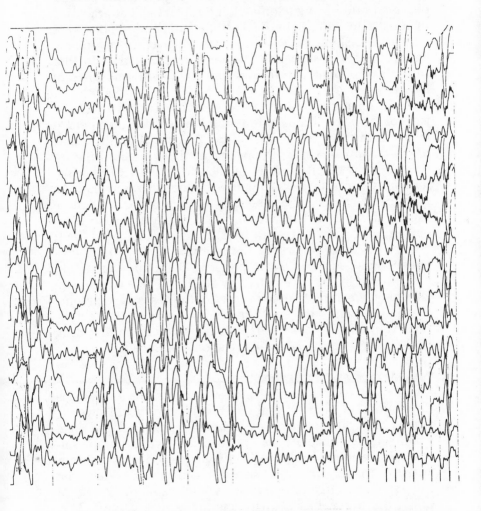

his brother collect hay. While he was holding a bale of oat hay, his arms jerked upward, flipping him in backward-somersault fashion over several other bales. Fortunately, the guardrail kept him in the truck. A few days later his parents observed him having a tonic-clonic seizure just after getting up in the morning. His EEG showed multiple spike wave bursts consistent with a diagnosis of juvenile myoclonic epilepsy. After five years on Dilantin, he has had no further seizures and regularly throws around 150-pound bales of hay.

Juvenile myoclonic epilepsy usually starts with small jerks of the upper limbs or limbs and torso just after a person arises in the morning. Some of my patients describe a hair brush or cup of coffee flying out of their hands. When a limited number of neurons in the motor cortex discharge randomly, muscle jerks called myoclonic jerks occur. As more neurons discharge, the myoclonic jerks become more severe. If most of the neurons in the brain discharge, a person will have a generalized tonic-clonic (grand mal) seizure just after arising in the morning. This type of epilepsy begins most often at puberty. Symptoms are often precipitated by lack of sleep or by alcohol. There is a genetic tendency, meaning that 40 percent of the cases have parents or relatives who also could be diagnosed with this condition. Valproate (Depakote) is now considered the first drug of choice in treating juvenile myoclonic epilepsy.

PARTIAL (FOCAL) EPILEPSIES
Some people have a small area of brain damage that has little effect on their normal day-to-day activities. However, when brain cells discharge excessively in that damaged area, small seizures occur. These seizures are called partial seizures. If the excessive brain discharge spreads to affect other areas of the brain larger seizures can occur. When the excessive discharge affects enough neurons on both sides of the brain, a generalized tonic-clonic seizure occurs. This type of seizure is called a secondarily generalized tonic-clonic seizure. In talking with my patients, I liken this

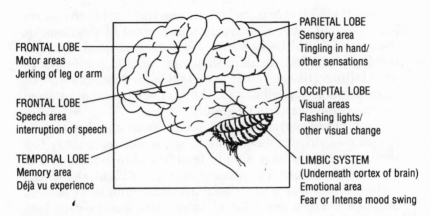

FRONTAL LOBE
Motor areas
Jerking of leg or arm

FRONTAL LOBE
Speech area
interruption of speech

TEMPORAL LOBE
Memory area
Déjà vu experience

PARIETAL LOBE
Sensory area
Tingling in hand/
other sensations

OCCIPITAL LOBE
Visual areas
Flashing lights/
other visual change

LIMBIC SYSTEM
(Underneath cortex of brain)
Emotional area
Fear or Intense mood swing

FIGURE 5.
A view of the lateral cortex of the brain.

occurrence to a short circuit in a wire throwing off sparks. If the sparks move along the wire far enough, a fuse blows and the power goes out.

Simple Partial Seizures. These include any small seizures that do not result in alteration of awareness. If the brain damage is in the motor area of the brain, the small seizure consists of jerking or stiffening in some part of the body. When the sensory area of the brain is damaged, a person will feel weird crawling or tingling sensations in some part of the body. Damage to the visual area results in flashing lights, colorful images, or other visual aberrations. Figure 5 shows a picture of the brain, naming the lobes of the brain and the function that each lobe serves. Damage to a particular area of the brain results in an exaggeration of the normal activity of that area of the brain.

I saw a boy, Sean, recently in my office who told me that he appeared to be asking questions in class without meaning to. He would suddenly turn his head to the left and raise his left arm. After a few seconds he would relax. His parents had noticed a few months earlier that his eyes had a tendency to go to the left and stay there a while. Sean had fallen off his bicycle once because he was unable to control his left-sided movement. Fortunately, most of the time his friends at school helped him when they noticed his head turning to the left. Usually they were able to prevent Sean from falling. His examination and all tests were normal. The history was so typical of partial motor seizures that I started him on carbamazepine (Tegretol).

Sometimes partial seizures result in an inability to talk. A middle-aged secretary came to see me because every few weeks she would have an odd feeling and be unable to talk for a minute. When it happened during the night, she would motion to her husband to hold her until symptoms passed. She had been under a lot of stress. Her examination was normal, but her EEG showed intermittent sharp waves over her left speech area. She developed a rash on carbamazepine, so I placed her on phenytoin. I also asked her to key in on ways that family stress triggered her symptoms.

A retired engineer came to see me because he experienced brief episodes of tingling of his left side every day. He had had a small stroke two months before that had caused his left side to be numb for six weeks. Extensive tests had shown no abnormalities of his blood pressure, heart, or blood vessels. The symptoms seemed characteristic of partial sensory seizures. Phenytoin reduced his symptoms by about 75 percent. After he was reassured by my diagnosis, and an explanation of its benign nature, he was able to resume his hobbies of golf, fishing, and saxophone playing.

Complex Partial Seizures. These are caused by damage to the temporal lobe or the frontal lobe of the brain. Dr. William Lennox, a pioneer in diagnosis and treatment of epilepsy, referred to these seizures as psychomotor seizures because they involve a loss of awareness (*psycho*) and motor activity such as facial grimacing or repetitive mouth or hand movements (*motor*).

The temporal and frontal lobes of the brain are directly connected to the limbic area of the brain. The limbic area is called the primitive brain because it appeared early in the evolution of the brain and regulates emotion. Because the temporal and frontal lobes connect directly with the limbic area, changes in feeling states—especially fear—may be associated with complex partial seizures.

Memory is stored in the temporal lobes. Disturbances in temporal lobe function may result in the frequent experience of déjà vu, the sensation of having experienced something before. Less often a person will not recognize familiar surroundings or circumstances, an experience called jamais vu. Many patients have difficulty with their memory. Some experience the feeling of being disconnected from their body or floating off.

The frontal lobes are involved in planning activities and strategies. Damage to the frontal lobes may cause slowing of decision making, or slowing of mental and motor activities. If the underside of the frontal lobe (orbito-frontal area) is damaged, seizures may be preceded by an odd, usually unpleasant, smell.

Complex partial seizures are caused by damage to a small part of the temporal or frontal lobe of the brain. They result in overexcitation of neurons in the damaged region. If the overexcitation remains confined to a very small area, an isolated experience of déjà vu, vertigo, fear, or odd smell may occur. This occurrence is known as an *aura*. When the area of overexcitation spreads to adjacent regions of the temporal or frontal lobe, a complex partial seizure occurs. If the excessive electrical discharge spreads from the temporal or frontal lobe to involve a large part of both sides of the brain, a generalized tonic-clonic seizure (grand mal) results.

Imagine the turmoil Dale, a nineteen-year-old patient, experienced after he had his first tonic-clonic seizure while he was watching television with his girlfriend. That seizure was preceded by an unpleasant smell of burning rubber. He had no more tonic-clonic seizures after starting phenytoin (Dilantin). Instead he had repeated auras consisting of the smell of burning rubber, often with a simultaneous sensation of floating out of his chair. After some of these auras he would lose awareness and his body would twist. Because of the seizures, Dale quit college, stopped dating, and went to live with his parents. His complex partial seizures occurred frequently despite the addition and substitution of different medications. He was one of the first patients to enter into a comprehensive biofeedback and counseling program with my associate Donna Andrews. After learning to control his seizures totally, Dale finished college, married, and became a successful business professional.

Susan has not yet reached her goal of total seizure control. Now in her twenties, she has had complex partial seizures since early childhood. Choice of medication has been limited because both carbamazepine and phenytoin

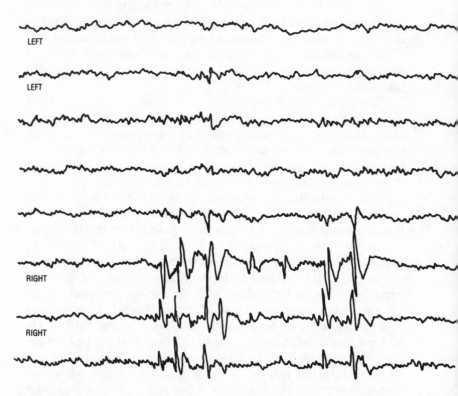

FIGURE 6.
Twenty-five-year-old man with complex partial seizures with spike abnormality over right side of brain.

lowered her blood count. When I saw her initially, she seemed overdrugged and drowsy on a combination of valproate and primidone. More than ten times every month, she would have an odd feeling followed by a loss of awareness of her surroundings of several minutes' duration. Work was a difficult chore and she hadn't been able to attend school. With our counseling and biofeedback approach, she was able to reduce her medication substantially. She continues to average three complex partial seizures per month. Nonetheless, she holds a full-time job while keeping up with a rigorous schedule of night classes. Her biggest disappointment is that because of incomplete seizure control, she cannot yet obtain a driver's license.

Complex partial epilepsy is the most difficult form of epilepsy to control with medications, probably because the temporal and frontal lobes perform the complicated brain functions that make us human. I urge people with complex partial epilepsy to consider the counseling and biofeedback approach described in other chapters of this book.

Less Common Forms of Epilepsy. Some forms of epilepsy are common in infancy and early childhood. Since this book emphasizes self-management techniques, I have left these types out of my discussion. Infantile spasms, Lennox-Gastaut syndrome, and seizures associated with degenerative neurological diseases occur with sufficient frequency that you may want more information on them. I suggest that you ask a pediatric neurologist to recommend some good textbooks on pediatric epilepsy.

In your notebook:

- If you know what type of epileptic seizure you have, describe it. You may have more than one.
- Find your type in the descriptions given in this chapter and read about it again carefully. Explain whether or not your seizures fit the above description exactly or if they vary. (If your type is rare, your neurologist can suggest further reading.)
- If possible, identify your type of physical preseizure aura by looking at figure 5. Describe how your aura experience is the same or different from the typical ones described therein.

4

Medical Technology and the Diagnosis of Epilepsy

The initial step in investigating a case of epilepsy is a full history, from both the patient and a witness, and clinical examination . . . the neurologist, with his clinical neurophysiological (EEG) and neuroradiological (x-ray) colleagues is best equipped to undertake the initial evaluation of patients suspected of epilepsy, and from his experience can offer useful advice . . . particularly on treatment.

—Dr. C. Marsden and Dr. E. H. Reynolds[1]

I interned at San Francisco General Hospital in 1967, the year that was also "the summer of love." At that time neurological diagnostic tests were crude if not brutal. In fact, the need to perform one of those tests called a pneumoencephalogram almost kept me from becoming a neurologist. The great American neurosurgeon William Dandy had introduced the pneumoencephalogram, also known as a PEG, in 1918. The PEG was performed by injecting air through a spinal needle inserted into the lower back. The air then made its way into the spinal fluid cavities of the brain. X-rays of the skull with this air in the ventricles demonstrated distortions of them or enlargement of the spinal fluid spaces. The PEG allowed doctors to diagnose tumors or brain atrophy. But these diagnostic advantages were offset by serious disadvantages: Patients experienced pain during the procedure and afterward suffered excruciating headaches.

Only twenty years have passed since my neurological residency. In 1968, at the University of California, San

43

Francisco, we performed PEG and arteriogram tests on many patients with unexplained onset of seizures. Yet, I'm thankful to say, the PEG is now as extinct as the dinosaur. We now have comfortable testing. In the early 1970s, computerized axial tomograph (CAT or CT) was developed to allow doctors to obtain pictures of the brain itself. The first scanners were called EMI scanners after the Beatle musicians' record company that financially supported early research and development. Subsequent CAT or CT scanners with increased sensitivity allow accurate diagnosis of tumors, strokes, and brain atrophy.

The first CAT scan in Santa Rosa was performed in 1975 on a sixteen-year-old patient of mine with sudden headache and coma. Michael's scan showed bleeding deep in his left parietal brain area. Fortunately, he began to recover and a series of scans allowed us to see that his bleeding had stopped spontaneously without surgery. A few years later, he began to have seizures caused by residual damage in the same left parietal area of the brain. Medication controlled the seizures. After graduating from college, Michael is now a successful businessman.

The PEG was not only extremely painful; it was often inaccurate. In 1976, I was asked to consult on a twenty-two-year-old man, Jimmie, who was then hospitalized at a state hospital. He experienced frequent complex partial seizures as well as behavioral problems. Doctors at a university medical center had attributed his seizures to an anomaly of his brain seen on a PEG test. A few years ago Jimmie left the state hospital and moved in with his mother in Santa Rosa. He came to see me because of persistent seizures on high doses of medication. I tested him with a CT scan, which was perfectly normal, as it is for most people with seizures. Knowing he didn't have a brain anomaly made a difference to him, his motivation, and his supervisor at the structured workshop where he works. Recently this supervisor started to work with Jimmie using counseling and biofeedback techniques. His seizures decreased, from five to ten a day to just a few per week. Even more impressive, he now helps support his mother with his earnings.

Doctors who thought they were on a different planet with the CT scan never dreamed that they would take a journey to another galaxy just ten years later. Soon after the CT scan was introduced, researchers set to work to develop an entirely new technology known as *magnetic resonance imaging (MRI)*. This technology combines physicists' basic discoveries of the 1950s with the exploding revolution in computer sciences. It uses a giant magnet and sound waves to take pictures with no x-ray radiation. The magnetic resonance or MRI scan gives a picture of the brain in anatomic detail. Tiny areas of brain atrophy, tumor, or blood vessel irregularities called vascular anomalies are now visible.

Last month I saw Betty, a thirty-six-year-old hairdresser who was having repeated unpleasant tingling and burning sensations in the left side of her face. The sensations occurred ten or twenty times an hour, and lasted ten seconds or less. They frightened her so much that she went to an emergency room on a Saturday night. The emergency room doctor ordered a CT brain scan that was read as normal. I saw Betty a few days later and thought that her symptoms were serious enough to warrant a magnetic resonance scan despite the added expense. Sure enough, the MRI scan showed a distinct tumor in the temporoparietal area of the brain. The tumor was successfully treated with surgery and radiation, but she began to have partial seizures after the surgery, I prescribed carbamazepine for her seizures.

The new sophisticated CT and MRI scanners have made my patients' lives and my life as a neurologist much more pleasant. When patients develop seizures, I no longer have to perform painful and inaccurate tests to exclude tumors or blood vessel malformations as causes. However, most seizure patients I see have normal CT and MRI scans. Less than 10 percent of adults with epilepsy have tumors, blood vessel anomalies, or other abnormalities on their brain scans. An even smaller percentage of children with seizures have tumors, blood vessel anomalies, or congenital anomalies. The scans allow me to recommend appropriate treatment to the minority of patients with brain abnormalities. Even more important, I can reassure the vast majority of my patients with epilepsy that the structure of their brain is perfectly normal. Their sigh of relief is music to my ears!

Many of my patients ask, "If my brain scan is normal, why do I have seizures?" I don't have a definitive answer. Generalized epilepsy is probably caused by an imbalance of chemicals in the brain, called *neurotransmitters*. Scientists have discovered many neurotransmitters, such as acetylcholine, norepinephrine, dopamine, N-methyl-D-aspartate, and gamma aminobutyric acid, which the brain needs to function normally. They do not yet understand the ways in which an imbalance of these chemicals causes seizures. On the other hand, partial epilepsy is often caused by microscopic damage to the brain that is too small to be detected by the naked eye or the computers that process CT and MRI scan data. When my patients' brain scans are normal, I base my diagnosis of epilepsy on the history of repeated seizures.

Neurologists call epilepsy with a known cause *symptomatic* or *secondary* epilepsy. Secondary epilepsies include those due to tumors, strokes, brain hemorrhage, or infections. Epilepsy of unknown cause is termed *idiopathic* or *primary* epilepsy. I tell my patients, "That means I don't know the cause and, therefore, I'm the idiot in the word *idiopathic*." I believe medical science is on the threshold of exciting discoveries that will determine many of the causes of idiopathic epilepsy. New techniques in neurochemistry, neurophysiology, and molecular engineering will unlock the biological secrets of this ancient malady.

As compared to CT and MRI scans, the electroencephalogram (described in chapter 3) picks up abnormalities in patients with epilepsy more frequently. About 75 percent of my patients with epilepsy have abnormalities in their EEGs. A single EEG may be normal, but repeating the EEG several times allows me to see irregularities in the brain's electrical activity. For complex partial epilepsy, abnormalities show up more often when a patient stays up for much of the night before the EEG is obtained. This test is called a sleep-deprivation EEG. In absence (petit mal) epilepsy, abnormalities can be produced by asking a person to overbreathe (hyperventilate). The EEG is very sensitive to body movement, eye blinking, or jaw clenching. These movements produce false irregularities, called *artifacts*, which obscure the actual brain wave pattern. Sometimes I have to be very crafty to differentiate true abnormalities from artifacts! Young children may require drugs to sedate them before an EEG, so that they stay quiet enough for the test to be readable.

A fifty-five-year-old plumber's history and his wife's description of his symptoms presented me with a diagnostic puzzle. Eugene would appear blank and pale to his wife during conversations and not respond to her questions. Did he have epilepsy? Or was the suffering from repeated tiny stroke-like symptoms, called *transient ischemic attacks,* which occur when oxygen doesn't reach some parts of the brain? It also occurred to me that he might be going deaf. Or, maybe this behavior was his way of taking mini-vacations from his wife!

Eugene's routine EEG was normal. When his symptoms became more frequent. I sent him to the EEG lab where the technician applied eight electrodes to his scalp. The electrodes were attached to a Walkman-sized recorder that he wore attached to his belt. After twenty-four hours, a cassette was removed from the recorder. When the cassette was analyzed on a monitoring screen, the EEG pattern showed frequent sharp waves over his right temporal brain region. The abnormality I saw in his twenty-four-hour ambulatory EEG was consistent with a diagnosis of complex partial epilepsy. After he started to take phenytoin (Dilantin) his spells became less frequent. Eugene's case is useful because it shows how longer EEG monitoring can help diagnose subtle symptoms of epilepsy.

The twenty-four-hour ambulatory EEG can demonstrate, as well, that some fading-out spells are not caused by epilepsy. Elizabeth, an eighty-year-old retired teacher, had been treated with different seizure medications. Several times each day she suddenly seemed "not to be there." A routine EEG had shown abnormal slow activity over both temporal lobes of her brain. I sent her to have a twenty-four-hour ambulatory EEG test, during which she had several lapses.

Since in this test one of the electrodes is attached to the chest wall, we could monitor heart activity in addition to her brain waves. Each time she had a mental lapse, there was a long pause in her heart activity. At those moments the heart simply wasn't pumping enough blood to her brain to keep her alert. Her diagnosis was heart block rather than epilepsy! All of her lapses stopped when she received a heart pacemaker.

A small number of people with epilepsy need even more sophisticated EEG monitoring, which is available at epilepsy centers. Closed-circuit television (CCTV) monitoring while a patient is staying in the hospital is useful for diagnosing people with frequent seizures who do not respond to treatment with several different drugs. Their histories and EEGs leave major questions about diagnosis. By monitoring their activity and EEG continuously on a closed-circuit television, the seizures can be correlated directly with their EEG over a period of days. Frequently the type of epileptic seizure becomes obvious after CCTV monitoring. Sometimes a patient has episodes that look like seizures, but has a normal EEG at the same time the episodes occur. This type of seizure is called a *pseudoseizure* because it is not caused by the abnormal discharge of neurons in the brain.

Severe emotional problems are the most common cause of pseudoseizures. During a vacation last year, my friend Dr. Gary Franklin recalled one of my first patients with pseudoseizures. A thirty-eight-year-old woman had been air transported the 300 miles from Eureka to San Francisco General Hospital because of continuous seizures. She had received large amounts of intravenous anticonvulsant medications. Nonetheless, she continued to have episodes that looked like seizures. It was 10 P.M. and I couldn't get an EEG right away. With Gary and an entourage of medical students and nurses looking on, I sat down on the patient's bed. Holding her hand, I asked, "What's wrong?" Out of her drug-induced stupor she tearfully replied, "My husband left me!" Gary asked me how I'd known that she wasn't having epileptic seizures. I told him that I didn't know, but that something didn't make sense, so I decided to explore another avenue.

Most patients I see for seizures recover quickly and resume their normal activities within minutes to hours. People with acute bacterial meningitis or viral encephalitis are a distinct exception. Last year I consulted at a rural hospital on a successful fifty-five-year-old woman who had her first generalized tonic-clonic seizure three days before. Mimi was hospitalized overnight, underwent normal CT brain scan and EEG tests, and went home taking Dilantin. She had a minimal fever of 99 degrees F while at the hospital.

The day I saw Mimi she developed a fever of 102 degrees F, had frequent lapses of attention, and then another generalized seizure. On examination she was mildly disoriented and drooled slightly from the left side of her mouth. I performed a spinal tap by inserting a needle into the lower back to remove spinal fluid. The spinal fluid showed abnormal white cells and an elevated protein level that was typical of viral encephalitis, an inflammation of brain tissue caused by infection with a virus. Because viral encephalitis can cause severe brain damage when it is caused by the herpes simplex virus, I treated her with acyclovir, a drug that is effective against herpes simplex virus when given intravenously. Her eventual total recovery was due to providence alone since her encephalitis turned out to be due to a different virus. Several months later she was back to her busy business schedule. Her EEG showed remnants of seizure activity, which led me to keep her on anticonvulsant medication for a period of time.

Several years ago, a mother brought her nineteen-year-old daughter to see me. Jackie had recently been hospitalized for six months with herpes encephalitis, an inflammation of the brain caused by the herpes simplex virus. Jackie was having frequent complex partial seizures, was unable to express herself, and was acting belligerent at home. I adjusted her seizure medication, and recommended that she have speech and occupational therapy. Frankly, I held little hope for this tragic young woman. Two years later, an attractive young woman stopped by my office to thank me for my help. Out of courtesy, I nodded when she asked if I remembered her. Only after she recounted her story did I recall that she was the same young woman who had been so neurologically devastated. Now she was enrolled in college! Equally amazing, Jackie was helping her boyfriend, another patient of mine, cope with and learn to reduce the frequency of his complex partial seizures.

Seizures occur commonly in people who have bacterial meningitis, an infection of the *meninges*, the membranes that cover the brain, caused by bacteria. Fever and stiff neck are clues to diagnosis. An immediate spinal tap, in which the physician inserts a needle into the lower back to withdraw samples of spinal fluid, tells the doctor what bug is causing the meningitis. Laboratory tests on the spinal fluid can identify the type of bacteria, as well as which antibiotic drugs will be effective in treating it. The doctor can then start massive amounts of the correct intravenous antibiotic. Prompt treatment of bacterial meningitis with antibiotics usually results in rapid cure.

A few years after I was in practice, Joe, a tough fifty-year-old laborer, approached me in my waiting room. "I just wanted to shake the hand of the man who saved my life," he said. Several months before, he was admitted to the hospital with frequent generalized tonic-clonic seizures, a high fever, and a stiff neck. His spinal tap showed many pneumococcus bacteria. Huge amounts of penicillin were started intravenously to kill the bugs along with Dilantin to stop his seizures. After a rocky hospital course, Joe made a complete recovery.

With bacterial meningitis, a few hours' delay in treatment can make the difference between total recovery and devastating brain damage. Thus, doctors perform spinal taps on infants and young children who have seizures associated with high fevers. Luckily most of these children do not have meningitis. Instead, they have a tendency—which sometimes runs in families—to seizures any time an ear infection or flu causes their temperature to rise suddenly over 103 degrees F. This condition, called *febrile seizures*, stops for most children after age five.

EEG tests are normal for children with febrile seizures.

Fevers can be brought down with sponge baths and acetaminophen (Tylenol), given orally or rectally. Unless high fevers with seizures occur frequently, doctors don't prescribe anticonvulsant medication. Some pediatricians teach parents how to give rectal anticonvulsant suppositories to prevent seizures whenever a child prone to febrile seizures develops a high temperature. For children who have seizures without fever, or abnormal EEG tests, doctors prescribe regular anticonvulsant medication.

What about treatment of epilepsy? Most people with epilepsy are helped by anticonvulsant medication when they take it over a long period of time. (I discuss many aspects of drug treatment in chapter 5.) Some people continue to experience frequent, disabling seizures despite trials of different antiepileptic medications, which is why I have helped to develop, with my colleague epilepsy counselor Donna Andrews, a comprehensive behavioral approach for people with epilepsy. Over fifteen years of practice, almost all of my patients who have chosen to try a behavioral treatment approach have experienced reduction in seizure frequency and enhanced quality of life. Therefore, I strongly recommend this approach to you and to anyone who continues to have seizures or difficulty coping with epilepsy. In recommending this approach, I differ from the majority of my neurological colleagues. Adrienne Richard eloquently explores the many aspects of a comprehensive behavioral approach to treatment of epilepsy in other chapters of this book. Chapter 6 discusses many of the reasons I believe in this new approach. In the remainder of this chapter, I will give equal time to the vast numbers of my colleagues who support a surgical approach for people with difficult types of epilepsy.

In the past fifteen years, neurosurgeons and neurologists have increasingly recommended surgical removal of abnormal temporal lobe brain tissue for people with uncontrolled complex partial epilepsy. This type of brain surgery is not new. In the 1930s, at the Montreal Neurological Institute, Dr. Wilder Penfield surgically removed part or all of the temporal lobe of patients who had uncontrolled temporal lobe seizures. Penfield and others showed that memory problems remained mild following removal of extensive portions of one temporal lobe.[2, 3]

In contrast, an American neurosurgeon named Scofield produced total inability to encode memory when he removed the front section of both temporal lobes from a patient. Scofield's patient is still alive thirty years later and has been interviewed on a television special on the neurology of memory. Further research demonstrated that if a large portion of one temporal lobe was removed and the remaining temporal lobe contained significant damage, serious memory deficits would result. Although some individuals benefited from epilepsy surgery, others developed behavioral or neurological problems. Therefore, for some years, brain surgery for epilepsy went out of favor.

Depth electrode studies developed in the past fifteen years have allowed doctors to locate with better accuracy abnormal brain tissue that causes epilepsy. With the aid of computer-assisted scans, neurosurgeons place electrodes directly into areas of the brain from which epileptic activity is thought to originate. Continuous EEG recordings are obtained for days to weeks by connecting these electrodes to closed-circuit television EEG monitoring units. If the abnormal EEG activity can be localized to part of one temporal lobe, and the patient's seizures are consistent with the depth electrode studies, the patient may be referred for temporal lobe surgery. To be considered for surgery, the abnormal EEG activity must be present on only one side of the brain.

New stereotactic techniques, in which a needle is guided into the brain through a small hole in the skull using computer-assisted scanners, allow neurosurgeons to remove exceedingly small areas of brain. I had been under the impression that neurosurgeons could remove very small areas of a temporal lobe to control seizures. However, I learned otherwise when I attended the 1988 meeting of the American Epilepsy Society, which was devoted to surgical treatment of epilepsy. At this meeting many distinguished neurosurgeons and neurologists reported that large portions of the temporal lobe had to be removed to obtain good control of seizures. Nonetheless, they claimed that most of their patients had marked reduction in seizure frequency without increased problems with their memory.

Brain surgery for types of epilepsy caused by damage to areas of the brain other than temporal lobe remains more controversial. Sometimes scar tissue in one of the frontal lobes causes complex partial seizures. Neurosurgeons report inconsistent results in studies of surgical removal of frontal lobe tissue for control of seizures. Radical neurosurgical procedures have been used in children who have many seizures each day that interfere drastically with normal activities. When these seizures are caused by severe damage to one hemisphere of the brain with total paralysis of the opposite side of the body, neurosurgeons have removed an entire side of the brain. In other children, corpus callosum fibers that connect the right and left hemispheres of the brain have been cut to prevent a severe form of seizures—called drop seizures—where patients fall to the ground without warning and often injure themselves.

In my opinion, the place for surgery in treatment of epilepsy is more limited than my colleagues propose. Medical treatments have traditionally been limited by the extent of our knowledge. I urge that the surgical risks to existing brain function including speech, memory, and personality be weighed carefully against possible benefits.

Medical treatment of epilepsy has focused little attention on diet. In the 1950s, infant formula deficient in vitamin B_6 was proven to be the cause of an outbreak of seizures in a pediatric nursery. Later a small number of newborn babies with seizures, who were receiving a normal amount of vitamin B_6 in their formula, stopped having seizures after they were given extra doses of the vitamin. Rare amino acid deficiencies have been shown to cause seizures in certain infants and children. I think these conditions indicate the need for medical researchers to look more closely into the possible role that dietary factors, such as vitamins and amino acids, could play in prevention of seizures.

The human brain is an incredibly complex and amazing organ. Epilepsy is a symptom of disorder within the human brain. Yet it is up to the human brain to unravel the mysteries that cause epilepsy. Diagnostic testing—including the EEG, CT scan, and MRI scan—has come a long way toward giving us information about brain abnormalities that cause epilepsy. New techniques such as position emission tomography (PET) scanning and computerized EEG promise to give us more information. But we are a long way from knowing what actually causes epilepsy.

Remember that the disorder that causes epilepsy is there all the time, but the seizures are not. If you have epilepsy don't focus on the fact that you have a brain disorder. Instead marvel at the way your brain and body work harmoniously to create order. This way of looking at your brain will help you, as you learn more about the new approach to epilepsy developed in this book.

In your notebook:

• What diagnostic tests have you gone through?
• What did they reveal?
• Did they confirm what your doctor suspected already?
• Did they reveal something new?
• Were they inconclusive? For example, the EEG may or may not show abnormal brain waves.

5

Antiepileptic Drugs

Finally, it is important to remember that the goal of treat-
ment is to assist patients in their efforts to overcome . . .
the consequences of epilepsy. This means that treatment
consists of things done in collaboration with patients
rather than to or for them. . . . patients must be encouraged
to accept the ultimate responsibility for what they will let
the epilepsy do to their lives. It is simply a question of
this: Who will be the master, the patient or the epilepsy?

—Dr. Francis Forster and Dr. Harold Booker[1]

Anyone who has taken an antibiotic for a minor
infection three times a day for ten days knows how difficult
it is to remember every dose. Parents cringe at the thought
of making a child take a course of antibiotics. Imagine facing
that burden every day of your life!

If you have had seizures, chances are your doctor already
has put you on *antiepileptic drugs*. These drugs are also
called *anticonvulsants*. You probably already realize that
this treatment is a commitment to years of taking medication
at regular times every single day. What you may not know is
that before making this commitment, you have to make a
decision. The first step in deciding about antiepileptic medication is to question whether it is necessary. Do you really
have epilepsy, or have you had a seizure for another reason?
Are your brief mental lapses convenient vacations from your
hectic life or are they complex partial seizures?

Suppose you had a busy week and you got only four
hours of sleep a night. On Friday night to wind down you
had three highballs at a party. Before you know it, you find
yourself in an emergency room. The doctor explains that

although your CAT scan and EEG are normal, he wants you to take three Dilantin capsules every night. Bewildered, you ask your husband for an explanation. He tells you that after the party you passed out, turned blue, and had a seizure. Would you follow the emergency room doctor's advice? Or would you seek an opinion from a neurologist?

In my two years as an army neurologist, I saw seven enlisted men who had seizures in the early morning hours after a week of guard duty. Surviving on three hours of sleep every night for a week had caused five of them to have seizures. Five of them didn't have epilepsy: They had a low seizure threshold, which means they were more likely to have seizures when sleep deprived or severely stressed. I prescribed antiepileptic medication for only the two men who had epilepsy.

People whose first generalized seizure occurs after substantial loss of sleep, during a period of great stress, or after drinking a lot of alcohol may never have another seizure. I suggest that they modify their life habits instead of using antiepileptic medication. What if the seizure occurred without apparent precipitating cause? After a single seizure I can't predict the risk for further seizures. That is why I find it difficult to advise a person about use of antiepileptic medication after a first seizure.

A person with epilepsy is not allowed to drive unless seizures have been controlled for three to twelve months. Driving regulations vary from state to state. Antiepileptic medication reduces the likelihood of seizure recurrence. Faced with these facts, many adults choose to take antiepilepsy medication after even a single seizure. If driving were not an issue, I would advise patients to put off use of medication until they had two or more seizures. It makes sense for a person to know he is at risk for recurrent seizures before committing to long-term medication. Certainly for children under sixteen, it is wise to wait to prescribe medication until they have had two or more seizures.

When I prescribe antiepileptic drugs, I tell my patients that they must take the medication regularly. If they forget to take medication, I advise them to double the next dose.

Taking medication irregularly can increase the number and severity of seizures. If the dam that holds back a river to create a lake suddenly breaks, houses downstream will be flooded. Similarly when antiepileptic medication acts like a dam to hold excessive brain discharge in check, the brain rebounds with a huge discharge when medication is suddenly stopped. The result can often be a life-threatening condition called *status epilepticus.* A person in status epilepticus has seizure after seizure, without enough time in between to allow normal breathing and heart function.

One hundred years ago, neurologists would have regarded the antiepileptic medicines I prescribe routinely for my patients as miraculous wonder drugs. Examples from the past point out how drug treatment of epilepsy has improved in the twentieth century. Around 200 B.C., Serapion of Alexandria prescribed a drug for epilepsy "compounded from the excrement of a land crocodile, the heart and loins of a hare, and the blood of a sea turtle."[2] Dr. B. J. Wilder relates how doctors began to treat epilepsy with bromides in 1857 because they were used to prevent masturbation, which was thought to be the cause of epilepsy. Mark Twain disputed the effectiveness of bromides for his epileptic daughter. He wrote: "Jeanne, for whom there seemed to be no hope at all, stopped taking large doses of bromides. . . . and her attacks of petit mal had become less frequent."[3]

Yet in prescribing antiepileptic drugs, I feel as if I am walking a tightrope between stopping seizures and producing side effects. I must decide if potential side effects such as lowered blood count, liver damage, or drowsiness are outweighed by the benefits gained from controlling seizures. I still do not know how medications actually affect the cells in the brain to prevent seizures. Nonetheless, I know that antiepilepsy drugs are beneficial for most of my patients with epilepsy.

The modern era of drug treatment for epilepsy began when phenobarbital was introduced in 1912. In a quest for more effective epilepsy medicines, pharmaceutical companies soon developed other drugs that were chemically similar to phenobarbital. By the 1930s, Drs. Houston Merritt and

Tracy Putnam had developed an experimental animal model that could be used to test these drugs for effectiveness in blocking seizures. Two experimental models continue to be the major method for developing new drugs. In one model, experimenters give rodents a maximal electrical shock (MES) to produce seizures. Drugs that prevent MES seizures in the animal model usually are effective against human generalized tonic-clonic seizures. In the other model, experimenters give rodents the drug pentylenetetrazol (PTZ) to produce seizures. Drugs that prevent PTZ seizures in rats or mice are usually effective against absence seizures.

Phenytoin was the first effective anticonvulsant drug discovered by trial-and-error pharmaceutical research. It was introduced as Dilantin in 1938. Similar research produced two other drugs with similar chemistry: primidone (Mysoline) in 1954 and ethosuximide (Zarontin) in 1960. Other drugs have fallen by the wayside because of toxic side effects. Carbamazepine (Tegretol), introduced in the United States in 1974, and valproate (Depakote), introduced in 1978, are chemically different, although they were discovered by using the same experimental approach.

The fact that antiepileptic drugs have been discovered through trial-and-error pharmaceutical research may explain why they have so many serious side effects. Scientists are just beginning to understand how brain chemistry and physiology regulate normal brain function. I think that this understanding will eventually result in more specific and less toxic medications for epilepsy.

Neurologists have developed guidelines for prescribing antiepilepsy drugs. I will use the classification of seizure types described in chapter 3 to indicate the drug that is most likely to be effective. In the following description, the medications of first choice are italicized. *Phenytoin, carbamazepine, valproate,* phenobarbital, and primidone are effective against generalized tonic-clonic seizures. Absence seizures are reduced by *ethosuximide* and *valproate.* Partial seizures including complex partial seizures respond to *carbamazepine, phenytoin,* phenobarbital, primidone, and valproate. Myoclonic seizures are treated with *valproate,* acetazolamide, phenobarbital, and benzodiazepines. Less common types of seizures include infantile spasms treated with adrenocorticotropic hormone (ACTH) and cortisone, and Lennox-Gastaut syndrome in children variably responsive to a mixture of valproate and benzodiazepines. Table 1 lists indications for antiepileptic medications.

These medications have at least two names. I gave you the generic name, which usually describes something about

TABLE 1

Drug Information Chart

Antiepileptic Medication	*Types of Seizures Treated**
phenytoin (Dilantin)	Generalized: tonic-clonic, tonic, clonic; complex partial, simple partial
carbamazepine (Tegretol)	Generalized: tonic-clonic, tonic, clonic; complex partial, simple partial
phenobarbital	Generalized: tonic-clonic, tonic, clonic; simple partial, complex partial
sodium valproate (Depakote, Depakene)	Generalized: absence and tonic-clonic, myoclonic, atonic†
primidone (Mysoline)	Complex partial, simple partial
ethosuximide (Zarontin)	Absence
mephobarbital (Mebaral)	Similar to phenobarbital but causes less hyperactivity in some children
clonazepam (Klonopin)	Myoclonic, akinetic
acetazolamide (Diamox)	Myoclonic, complex partial

Source: Adapted from *Taking Control of Your Epilepsy: A Workbook for Patients and Professionals* with permission of Andrews-Reiter Epilepsy Project Inc.

*I have used the new classification terminology in these tables. Generalized tonic-clonic, tonic, and clonic = grand mal; absence = petit mal; complex partial = temporal lobe or psychomotor; simple partial = focal.

†Pending studies indicate that valproate is effective for complex partial seizures.

the drug's chemical composition. Acetaminophen and aspirin are examples of generic names. Drugs also have patented brand names, chosen by the drug companies to attract customers to use their drug. Tylenol, Ex-Lax, and Alka Seltzer are examples of brand names of nonepileptic drugs. When a pharmaceutical firm first discovers a new drug, it is marketed under its brand name. When the patent expires, different pharmaceutical companies then market the drug under its generic name. For example, phenytoin was initially marketed as Dilantin, carbamazepine was sold initially as Tegretol, and valproate was sold as Depakote. Generic drugs are usually significantly less expensive than brand-name drugs.

Is it better to pay more money for a brand-name drug? Questions have arisen about the reliability of generic versus brand-name antiepileptic drugs. Unreliable batches of generic phenytoin were marketed at one time. Different fillers and inactive ingredients can affect the body's response to generic drugs. For example, most generic antiepileptic drugs are absorbed into the bloodstream and eliminated more rapidly than the brand-name drug. The result is higher initial blood levels and lower levels several hours after the drug is taken.

Let's take the case of phenytoin. Medicines like phenytoin, which are taken only one or two times a day, are particularly affected by this difference in rate of absorption. Whereas Dilantin can be taken as a single daily dose, generic phenytoin must be taken in several smaller doses spaced throughout the day. If you change from a brand-name antiepileptic drug to a generic one, it is wise to ask your doctor to retest your blood level.

Another problem with generic drugs is that pharmacies may purchase them from different pharmaceutical companies. One month company X has a better price and the next month company Y is cheaper. The characteristics of a generic antiepileptic drug manufactured by company X may be different than company Y's drug. Ask your pharmacist if he keeps the same manufacturer for a particular generic drug.

In prescribing antiepileptic medications, I consider the age and sex of a patient. I don't like to use phenytoin in children since it can cause overgrowth of gums, coarsening of facial features, facial hair growth, or acne. Fatal liver damage has occurred in young children taking valproate. I shy away from using valproate for children under two years old or in people with a history of liver disease. Some people find it very difficult to take medication several times per day. Dilantin, which can be given as a single daily dose, is a more reliable medicine for them.

Every rule has exceptions. For example, I started a ten-year-old boy on valproate after he had severe generalized seizures. Frank's hair changed color and he gained a lot of weight, prompting me to change him to carbamazepine. When his white blood count fell too much, I placed him on phenytoin, which caused no significant side effects.

I don't like to prescribe valproate for patients with a history of liver problems. But Sue, a lovely twenty-five-year-old woman, was disabled by tonic-clonic seizures that occurred at least once each month. She developed an allergic skin rash on carbamazepine. Phenytoin caused an odd skin condition as well as abnormal elevation of liver enzymes, which meant her liver might sustain permanent damage from continuing that medicine. Liver tests were abnormal with primidone as well. Out of desperation, because I had exhausted other options, I placed her on valproate, even though her liver tests had been abnormal on two other medications. Sue has had no seizures for one year and her liver tests have remained normal.

A seventeen-year-old boy told me that he felt like a guinea pig because I kept changing his medication. John had daily tonic-clonic seizures that should have been controlled with valproate. Increasing the dose made him tired but didn't help his seizures. I switched him to phenytoin. After two weeks without seizures he broke out in a measles-like rash. He wanted to quit taking medicine and drop out of school. I talked him into trying one last medication. To our mutual relief, carbamazepine stopped his seizures with no ill effects.

The patients I described above developed intolerable side effects on several medications. I would have preferred not to prescribe medications for them at all. However, their seizures were severe enough to warrant trials of other antiepileptic medications. Fortunately, most of my patients do not develop severe side effects with antiepileptic drugs. Because the potential for damaging side effects exists, I monitor patients closely whenever I start them on a new medication.

What are the most common side effects of anticonvulsant medications? Two percent of patients develop a skin rash within days to weeks of taking carbamazepine, phenytoin, or phenobarbital. Fewer develop a rash with valproate. The skin rash indicates that a person is allergic to a medication and that more drastic damage will occur if they continue taking the medication. Whereas drug allergy usually is visible as a rash, other reactions to drugs can occur that produce invisible side effects. These harmful effects of drugs are called *toxicity*.

Potential toxicity is different for different drugs. For example, carbamazepine can cause a drop in the white blood cell count or red blood cell count. Valproate can damage the liver. Doctors can detect early evidence of toxicity by measuring a complete blood count (CBC) or liver enzymes. Luckily, signs of toxicity usually appear within a few months of starting a medication. Toxic side effects are completely reversible if the medication is stopped soon after they appear. I routinely order a CBC and liver function tests monthly for the first three months after I prescribe carbamazepine or valproate. If the tests are normal for the first three months, I increase the time interval between blood tests to every six months. Table 2 lists medications, potential toxicity, and monitoring tests commonly performed.

I believe that the most important reason to prescribe antiepileptic medication is to improve the quality of my patients' lives. The general rules I have outlined do not tell me how a particular person will respond to a medication. Whereas one patient may experience total control of seizures with a high dose of a medication, a second may respond to a low dose, and a third may obtain no benefit. I ask my patients to keep a daily record of the number and severity of their seizures. I welcome notes about any aspect of their daily lives that might be affected by medications, including

TABLE 2

Drug Information Chart

Antiepileptic Medication	Common Side Effects	Rare Side Effects*·**	Blood Tests to Monitor
phenytoin (Dilantin)	imbalance, double vision, confusion, gum overgrowth, body hair growth	neuropathy, liver damage, decreased white blood cell count	CBC, liver function tests
carbamazepine (Tegretol)	double vision, mental confusion	decreased blood count, bone marrow depression, liver damage	CBC, liver function tests
phenobarbital	drowsiness, memory loss child: hyperactivity		
sodium valproate (Depakene, Depakote)	weight gain, increased levels of other anticonvulsant drugs, hair loss	acute liver damage, decreased platelet count	liver function tests, serum ammonia level, platelet count
primidone (Mysoline)	drowsiness, memory loss, child: hyperactivity	bone marrow depression	CBC
ethosuximide (Zarontin)	nausea, loss of appetite, drowsiness	bone marrow depression	CBC
clonazepam (Klonopin)	drowsiness, imbalance		

Source: Adapted from *Taking Control of Your Epilepsy: A Workbook for Patients and Professionals* with permission of Andrews-Reiter Epilepsy Project Inc.

*Some individuals will just "not like" a particular drug. This feeling should be respected.

**Allergy may be seen with any drug. Allergy appears most often as a skin rash within days to a month.

level of alertness, sleep pattern, memory, and interactions with other people. My goal is for patients to have control of their seizures with no drug side effects. This goal usually means regulating the dosage so that they take the smallest amount of medication that will prevent seizures.

After antiepileptic drugs are absorbed into the bloodstream from the intestines, they are metabolized by the liver. *Metabolized* means they are broken down into smaller chemical compounds. The liver metabolizes different drugs at different speeds. Then these smaller compounds are eliminated from the body by the kidneys at different speeds. The time that it takes the body to eliminate half of the quantity of a drug is defined as the drug's *half-life*. The dosage of a drug is the amount prescribed and the number of times each day that a person must take the drug. The dosage is determined by the drug's half-life and the individual's response to a particular drug.

When a drug is metabolized and eliminated from the body quickly, it has a short half-life. Dosage of drugs with a short half-life such as carbamazepine and valproate must be divided so that they are taken in smaller amounts several times a day. If a drug is metabolized and eliminated from the body slowly, it has a long half-life. Drugs with a long half-life such as Dilantin and phenobarbital can be taken once a day because they remain active in the body for twenty-four hours (table 3).

A key reason that people respond differently to antiepileptic drugs is that they metabolize medication at different speeds. Several hours after taking the same dosage of medication, a person who metabolizes quickly will have less in his bloodstream than a person who metabolizes slowly. Therefore, a person who metabolizes a drug quickly will require a higher dosage of medication to obtain the same effect. I can't measure the rate of metabolism of my patients, but I can determine how much of an antiepileptic drug is in a person's blood. This test is called a *blood level*. Standard medical laboratories measure blood levels quickly and accurately. The purpose of getting a blood level is to check whether it is in the *therapeutic range*. The therapeutic range for each drug is the concentration below which the drug is

TABLE 3

Drug Information Chart

Antiepileptic Medication*	Dosage Range	Frequency of Dosage
phenytoin (Dilantin)	adult: 200–600 mg/day child: 10–30 mg/kg/day	1 time/day 1–2 times/day
carbamazepine (Tegretol)	adult: 400–1800 mg/day child: 10–30 mg/kg/day	2–3 times/day 2–4 times/day
phenobarbital	adult: 30–180 mg/day child: 2–6 mg/kg/day	1 time/day 1–2 times/day
sodium valproate (Depakote; Depakene)	adult: 750–3000 mg/day child: 20–50 mg/kg/day	2 times/day 2–4 times/day
primidone (Mysoline)	adult: 250–1000 mg/day child: 15–30 mg/kg/day	2–3 times/day 2–4 times/day
ethosuximide (Zarontin)	adult: 500–1500 mg/day child: 10–25 mg/kg/day	2 times/day 2–4 times/day
clonazepam (Klonopin)	1–10 mg/day	2–3 times/day
acetazolamide (Diamox)	adult: 250–1000 mg/day child: 125–500 mg/day	2 times/day 2–3 times/day

Source: Adapted from *Taking Control of Your Epilepsy: A Workbook for Patients and Professionals* with permission of Andrews-Reiter Epilepsy Project Inc.

*Listed under generic name with brand name in parentheses.

mg = milligram; mg/kg = milligram per kilogram; 1000 milligrams = 1 gram; 28.35 grams = 1 ounce; 1 kilogram = 2.2 pounds

not effective in preventing seizures and above which significant side effects occur (table 4).

Blood levels are more reliable indicators if they are measured before the next dose of medicine is due to be taken. Usually I recommend that my patients go to the lab in the morning, before the first dose of the day is taken. The goal is to achieve control of seizures with the lowest effective blood level of the drug. Side effects, especially drowsiness and difficulty in thinking, tend to increase as the blood level of a drug increases.

TABLE 4

Drug Information Chart

Antiepileptic Medication	Range of Therapeutic Levels*, **	Serum Half-Life	Time to Reach Steady Level after Starting Drug
phenytoin (Dilantin)	6-20 μg/ml	9-140 hours (24 hours)	7-21 days (5 days)
carbamazepine (Tegretol)	4-10 μg/ml	10-30 hours (12 hours)	5-10 days (3 days)
phenobarbital	10-40 μg/ml	adult: 50-160 hours child: 30-70 hours (4 days)	up to 30 days (3 weeks)
sodium valproate (Depakene, Depakote)	50-100 μg/ml	8-20 hours (12 hours)	4 days (3 days)
primidone (Mysoline)	5-15 μg/ml	4-12 hours (12 hours)	up to 30 days (3 days)
ethosuximide (Zarontin)	50-100 μg/ml	adult: 40-70 hours child: 20-40 hours (2 days)	14 days (10 days)
clonazepam (Klonopin)	??	20-60 hours	14 days

Resources for the chart: *First values: Laidlaw, J., and A. Richens, *A Textbook of Epilepsy*, Churchill Livingstone, London, 1982. **Second values (in parentheses): Porter, R., *Epilepsy: 100 Elementary Principles*, W. B. Saunders, London, 1984.

μg = microgram; ml = milliliter

Source: Tables 1–4 adapted from *Taking Control of Your Epilepsy: A Workbook for Patients and Professionals* with permission of Andrews-Reiter Epilepsy Project Inc.

As a resident in neurology, I was taught to prescribe several different drugs when seizures were not controlled with a single drug. I noticed that most patients on several antiepileptic drugs developed increased side effects, but continued to have seizures. Other neurologists noted similar problems with *polytherapy*, the practice of prescribing several antiepileptic drugs at once. Neurologists now favor *monotherapy*, the use of a single drug in treatment of epilepsy. Studies have demonstrated that polytherapy increases side effects of drugs, whereas seizure control is often not improved and sometimes worsens. For an occasional patient, use of two drugs at the same time can be helpful.

It is not always necessary to increase or change antiepileptic medication when a person has uncontrolled seizures. Many patients have improved control of their seizures by using techniques described in this book. Others have actually had fewer seizures when I reduced the dosage of their medication.

Rarely, people have other medical conditions that are contributing to seizures, even though on optimal medication. Jack developed generalized seizures from brain damage after falling from a high scaffolding. He underwent an operation to remove two-thirds of his stomach after the same accident. When I saw him for the first time, five years after the accident, he was taking two anticonvulsant drugs with poor seizure control. I ordered a glucose tolerance test that measures blood-sugar level for several hours after drinking a sugar-water solution. His sugar level after three hours was only 25, an extremely low level that can by itself cause seizures. Jack now eats six small meals a day to control hs blood-sugar level and takes a moderate dose of phenytoin. He has had no seizures for four years.

ANTIEPILEPTIC MEDICATION DURING PREGNANCY

When a pregnant woman has repeated generalized seizures, her baby may be damaged by lack of oxygen. If she falls during a seizure, the baby can be injured. Most women with epilepsy must take anticonvulsant medication during their pregnancies. The dilemma is that these medications can cause birth defects. Phenytoin has been shown to cause cleft lip and palate and heart defects at a rate two to three times higher than the general population. Valproate can cause a defect of the spine called spina bifida in 1 to 2 percent of babies whose mothers take the drug in the early stages of pregnancy. Two tests can detect if valproate has caused spina bifida in the unborn fetus. Abnormal levels of serum alpha-fetaprotein in a mother's blood in the first twenty weeks of her pregnancy may indicate her baby has spina bifida. During the fourth month, an ultrasound test of the fetus may reveal the same abnormality.

As I set out to write this book, carbamazepine (Tegretol) was considered the antiepileptic drug least likely to cause birth defects. However, in June 1989, Dr. Kenneth Lyons Jones and his colleagues published a study demonstrating that carbamazepine may be as likely to cause birth defects as phenytoin.[4] He and other researchers stress that the risk of birth defects is considerably greater if a woman takes two or more antiepileptic drugs during her pregnancy.[5]

If you are a woman who needs to take antiepileptic medications to prevent seizures, what should you do if you want to have a child? First, realize that the risk of having a child with birth defects caused by your antiepileptic drug is less than 6 percent; the risk of serious birth defects is less than 2 percent. Your odds of having a healthy child are very good. Discuss the risk of uncontrolled seizures harming you or your unborn child with your family doctor or obstetrician and your neurologist. If you have never had a generalized seizure, ask about the risk of not taking medication during your pregnancy. If you are taking more than one antiepileptic medication, could you change to taking only one before you plan to get pregnant? Remember that you should undertake any changes in your antiepileptic drug regimen *before* you plan to get pregnant! Once you are pregnant it is too late to contemplate changes because birth defects due to antiepileptic drugs occur early in pregnancy.

Blood levels of anticonvulsants tend to decrease during the fifth to seventh months of pregnancy, because a mother's blood volume and metabolism increase to provide nourishment to her growing baby. Women who have seizures when their medication drops below a moderate to high blood level may need to take more medication during this stage of pregnancy. If a pregnant woman's dosage is increased at this stage of pregnancy, it will need to be lowered after she has her baby. Can a mother who takes antiepileptic medication safely breast-feed her baby? In my opinion, the great benefits a baby and mother get from breast-feeding outweigh risks of the baby getting a small amount of an antiepileptic drug through breast milk. I advise each woman to discuss these important questions with the doctor she sees for monthly prenatal checkups and with her neurologist.

DRUG INTERACTIONS AND WITHDRAWAL

The effectiveness or toxicity of antiepileptic drugs can be altered when other drugs are taken at the same time, which may lead to increased or decreased concentrations of the antiepileptic drug in the bloodstream; or antiepileptic drugs may cause decreased absorption of other drugs from the gastrointestinal tract. Specific drug interactions may include reduction of antibiotic absorption necessitating higher doses of antibiotic; reduced effectiveness of oral contraceptives; reduced effectiveness of steroid agents or nonsteroidal anti-inflammatory drugs; and reduction of serum calcium and folic acid levels. I advise you to check with your doctor or pharmacist about possible drug interactions before starting any new medication.

People who take medication have a difficult decision to make after they have been seizure-free for several years. Several neurologists have reported in recent studies that up to 65 percent of people can go off medication without having seizures, if they have had no seizures for two to three years. Withdrawing antiepileptic medication without seizure recurrence is most successful among people who had few seizures before treatment began, whose seizures were easily controlled with low to moderate dosage of medication, and whose electroencephalograms were normal on medication.

TABLE 5

Drug Information Chart

New Antiepileptic Medication	Dosage Range	Frequency of Dosage	Types of Seizures Treated	Common Side Effects
gabapentin (Neurontin)	adult: 1,800–3,600 mg/day child: *	2 times/day	Complex partial**	sleepiness, imbalance, dizziness, fatigue AED (antiepileptic drug) interaction: none
lamogitrine (Lamictal)	adult: 200–500 mg/day child: *	2 times/day	Complex partial**, Lennox-Gastaut	rash, dizziness, sleepiness, double vision, imbalance; positive effect—increased sense of well-being AED interaction: increased epoxide
vigabatrin (Sabril)	adult: 1,500–4,000 mg/day child: 50–100 mg/kg/day	1–2 times/day 2 times/day	Complex partial**	drowsiness, dizziness, imbalance, headache, (less common: behavioral changes or psychosis) AED interaction: decreased phenytoin level
felbamate (Felbatol)	adult: 1,800–3,600 mg/day child: 15–45 mg/kg/day	2–3 times/day 3–4 times/day	Complex partial**, Lennox-Gastaut, atonic	insomnia, anorexia, nausea, weight loss, headache, (uncommon: aplastic anemia) AED interaction: increased phenytoin, valproate, and epoxide; decreased carbamazepine levels

This drug is under an FDA advisory; consult your physician.

*Prescribed for children, but dosage not yet definitely established.

**Includes secondarily generalized seizures.

Current clinical research suggests that these new antiepileptic drugs may increase seizure control when used as second drugs in polytherapy without substantially increasing side effects. Three of them—gabapentin (Neurontin), lamogitrine (Lamictal), and vigabatrin (Sabril)—are new to the United States but have been used in Europe together with older antiepileptic drugs as add-on drugs in polytherapy. Future research will determine if these new drugs are effective when used as single drugs in monotherapy.

On page 67 of this chapter I recommend monotherapy for most people taking antiepileptic medication. If you continue to have seizures with optimum adjustment of a single antiepileptic drug, first add the nonmedication methods described in other chapters of this book to your treatment regimen. If seizures remain out of control, discuss with your medical doctor adding one of the new antiepileptic drugs as a second medication. Then report both changes in seizure control and significant side effects to your doctor to determine if the combination of antiepileptic drugs is beneficial or troublesome.

Felbamate (Felbatol), released in the United States in 1993 for monotherapy or polytherapy, has been placed on FDA advisory for use with caution because of reports of potentially fatal aplastic anemia and liver failure.

The same studies showed that the likelihood of seizures after withdrawal of medication was greater for people who had many seizures before starting medication. Seizure recurrence was also more likely when it took several changes of medication and adjustment of dosages before seizure control was achieved, or when the EEG continued to show a seizure pattern on medication. People with generalized seizures were more successful in going off medication without seizure recurrence than those with complex partial epilepsy. Neurologists advise people who decide to stop taking antiepileptic medication to taper the dosage slowly over a three- to twelve-month period.

Adrienne Richard describes her experience with medication in other chapters. She relates that medication caused her more problems than the actual seizures. I have many patients with similar experiences, who would rather risk a rare seizure than feel drowsy and think sluggishly. For other patients, the decision to use medication came after a long struggle. They prefer to continue with medication rather than rock the boat.

Everybody with epilepsy, at various stages of their lives, needs to make a personal decision about the use of antiepileptic drugs. To do so, he or she must ask the essential question: "Is my life better taking medication or would I do better without it?" I caution you to discuss the potential dangers of reducing antiepileptic medication with your doctor.

In your notebook:

- What medication or medications are you taking?
- What amounts (milligrams) do you take daily?
- Do you notice any side effects? (You may or may not.)
- Are you on several drugs? Since monotherapy is preferred today, ask your doctor to explain why he keeps you on several medications. Discuss one-drug therapy with him.

6

Toward a New Neurology

*Music has been a major part of Deborah Lee's life. But
when she walks to the podium to conduct the Santa Rosa
Symphony Orchestra at the June 11 Pops concert, it will be
more than a musical triumph.*

*Deborah is a soft-spoken woman of thirty-three, an
exotic-looking reflection of her Chinese-Swiss lineage. She
is bright and witty, unfailingly cheerful and fiercely independent. She has been in a wheelchair for thirteen years.*

*Deborah was a student at U. C. Davis, majoring in
preveterinary medicine, when she was injured in the crash
of a small aircraft in 1976. Damage to her brain affected
the use of muscles and nerves in her body and induced
epilepsy. Through the long years she has progressed from
immobility to semi-independence; from electric wheelchair to sports model, to standing upright in braces. None
of this could have been accomplished without many thousand pain-filled hours of rigorous therapy.*

*She gives speeches on the role of a handicapped person
living in an able-bodied world. The pops audience will
learn a mighty lesson on such matters when Deborah
stands before them, baton in hand. Her selection: the
happiest of tunes, Richard Rodgers' "Surrey with the
Fringe on Top."*

—Gaye LeBaron[1]

Debbie Lee was important in my life before I read
this news clip with my morning coffee on May 31, 1989.
Five years earlier she had appeared in my consultation room
for advice about her seizures. She experienced daily complex partial seizures despite high doses of two antiepileptic
drugs. I told her that she could control her seizures and
substantially reduce her medication. She would need to sail
into uncharted waters. I turned her over to my associate,
epilepsy counselor Donna Andrews, for the voyage.

On meeting Debbie, Donna said "I don't know why I'm saying this, but someday you are going to walk!" Donna's vision of Debbie proved correct. Within a few months her seizures were in control and she took only small doses of phenytoin. She can stand and has taken her first steps. She has written a book to help children control seizures. Debbie taught me never to underestimate my patients' potential for neurologic recovery.

It is not surprising that Donna Andrews would have had an expansive vision for Debbie Lee. Donna had been a whiz in high school, the type of kid who was always taking first place in science fairs. In her first year of premedical studies, she lapsed into coma. Generalized seizures followed. University neurologists diagnosed viral encephalitis. They predicted a dire outcome: probable institutional care. Ignoring this ominous prediction, Donna's parents took her home. She had frequent generalized and complex partial seizures despite high doses of medication. A severe allergy to one medication almost killed her.

Donna slowly recovered fragments of memory and reasoning ability. Yet, she continued to bump into things and fall down stairs because of frequent seizures. Then one day she had an awesome thought: "If the damage is there all the time, why aren't the seizures?" Neurologists still cannot answer that question. Neither can Donna, but she used that question to help her find a solution to her own disabling seizures. She began to observe herself all the time: between seizures, before seizures, and after seizures. She began to recognize similiar feelings that would precede all of her seizures. Next, she found that events in her life, including feelings of fear, worry, or anger or interactions with other people, would cause seizures. She called these events her "triggers." Identifying her triggers allowed her to reduce and eventually eliminate her seizures.

Control of seizures was the jumping-off point for Donna's remarkable neurological recovery. Donna raised three delightful and capable children. Doctors considered her youngest child, Charles, to be irreversibly handicapped after he had bacterial meningitis when he was three years old.

Donna didn't accept this bleak outlook. She started to teach Charles at home, as if he were an infant starting over again. He is now a handsome, intelligent college student. Her past accomplishments include work as Department of Health, Education, and Welfare epilepsy spokesperson, and as director of two major chapters of Epilepsy Foundation of America. She authored Project EASE, a major employment project for people with epilepsy. Donna subsequently obtained a master's degree in rehabilitation administration. She is completing work for a Ph.D. degree in psychology. However, the formal degrees are just the icing on the cake. The cake was created out of understanding learned by struggling with adversity.

Through chance and good fortune I met Donna Andrews in 1979. I had shared a train compartment with Dr. James Yandell on a glorious trip through China in 1978. The following year, Jim asked me to participate in teaching a biofeedback course that he and Dr. Ken Pelletier were directing. I included some thoughts on the use of biofeedback for people with epilepsy in my talk. Bursting with excitement, Donna confronted me after the lecture. She told me that I was the first neurologist she had met who seemed to understand that people had an ability to control their seizures. But, she told me, I underrated their ability.

I challenged Donna to prove that people with epilepsy could learn to control their seizures. She challenged me to help set up a pilot project with six of my patients whose seizures were out of control. Ray Lambert, a biofeedback whiz, clinical psychologist Dr. Al Kastl, and psychiatrist Dr. Sam Brown gave us assistance in setting up a pilot project. Donna worked each week with six of my patients. All of the patients had uncontrolled complex partial seizures, despite trials of several anticonvulsant medications. I had cared for each of the patients for at least two years. She taught them to observe events that triggered their seizures. They came to recognize feelings that preceded their seizures, termed the *preseizure aura*. In addition, she taught progressive relaxation and deep breathing exercises. Once they could relax, she taught them to control their brain wave patterns by using EEG biofeedback equipment.

After six months Donna said to me "I told you so." Five of the six patients had achieved dramatic control over their seizures. The one person who left the pilot project had limited ability to reason and remember. I concluded that people with reasonable ability to think and remember can learn to control their complex partial seizures. Donna dwelled instead on the one woman who left the pilot project. She concluded that we needed to learn more so that we could help that woman as well.

I admit that I get tired of being chided for my lack of bold vision. However, events have proven Donna's optimistic vision of people's inherent ability to help themselves to be correct. Sheila, a seemingly retarded woman in her twenties, was brought to the emergency room with generalized seizures at least once a month. Hearing of our project, Sheila's neurologist suggested that she work with Donna. One year later Sheila's mother, her neurologist, and even Donna were amazed. Not only had she learned to control her seizures but she had started to paint and already sold a few paintings.

Phyllis Grannis didn't want to give her eleven-year-old daughter antiepileptic medications. Heather had generalized tonic-clonic seizures, mostly at night. A very good pediatrician had prescribed phenobarbital. The first time I talked with Phyllis, I told her that Heather should take phenobarbital. Phyllis' intuition told her that there was a pattern to Heather's seizures. She wanted Heather to try to control her seizures without using medication. At her insistence, I agreed that Heather could work with Donna Andrews before starting antiepileptic medications.

Heather learned to identify events that seemed to precede her seizures the hard way. One seizure occurred six years later in high school. On the way home from a party, she was wondering about whether to kiss her date goodnight. Approaching the driveway of her house, she had a seizure. From this experience and others like it she learned that when she was nervous she tended to have more seizures. Her next step was to learn how to take care of herself when she was nervous so she wouldn't have a seizure. Now she feels confident on dates. She enjoys her pressured life as a college student and she hasn't had a seizure for two years.

After seeing Heather through the travails of epilepsy, Phyllis wanted to use what she had learned to help others. She donated her skills as a graphic artist to design and edit our workbook *Taking Control of Your Epilepsy: A Workbook for Patients and Professionals*. Then she decided to make a major career change: she gave up her successful graphic design business, studied with epilepsy counselor Donna Andrews, and completed a master's degree in counseling. She is now a remarkably effective epilepsy counselor in her own right with the Andrews-Reiter Epilepsy Project.

One of Phyllis' and Donna's joint accomplishments over the past two years has been their ground-breaking work with Darcy Fluitt. Darcy is a counselor in a structured workshop for developmentally disabled people that allows her to help clients with epilepsy every day they are at work. Many clients who were having frequent seizures, despite adjustments of antiepileptic medication, reduced the frequency of their seizures substantially in the workshop. Phyllis summarized how they achieve good results: "The key factors in success include presenting information concretely; repeating information many times; teaching abdominal breathing techniques with muscle and EEG biofeedback training; and most crucially, creating a supportive environment at home and work." She emphasized, in particular, "honoring and accepting the client as a unique expression of humanity and reinforcing the individual's belief in his or her ability, no matter how limited."

Sometimes I feel like a proud parent when I think of what my patients have accomplished. But, like a parent, I must remind myself that the accomplishments are the result of their own hard work, not mine. Sarah was the first patient with complex partial epilepsy I helped with counseling and biofeedback. Before having a seizure she would experience an intense feeling of "blue." She couldn't describe her aura any other way. Sarah's seizures diminished dramatically after she learned to key in on events that aggravated her. I was impressed by the mastery she gained over her seizures using deep-breathing exercises and biofeedback training. However, I really didn't understand her or her success until

I attended the opening of her first art show. There I gazed upon the most vivid abstractions of blue I had ever seen!

Other remarkable epilepsy patients come to mind: a woman who could barely care for herself, but who is now the proud and nurturing mother of two bouncy boys; another who has developed one of the most successful wineries in the county; several men, who as lads seemed too scattered to attend high school, but are now successful in their chosen professions. These people illustrate the "new neurology" better than anything I could write to describe it. They are a resounding positive answer to the question posed by Dr. William Lennox, who pioneered modern medical treatment of epilepsy: "Beyond the origin and mechanisms of seizures lie the subtle attributes and vicissitudes of each individual epileptic. What is his inward worth and stability when plagued by paroxysmal instability and when beset by secrecy and fear?"[2] Their inward worth and stability—women, men, boys, and girls—is as great as anyone else's. The new neurology seeks to assist every individual with epilepsy to reach his or her highest potential for fulfillment.

You might ask, "So this is just the good fortune of one doctor who happens to choose the right patients. Does it really apply to me or my loved one?" Yes, it very definitely applies to you and anyone who is willing to put the time and effort into taking control. To explain my bold statements, I'd like to draw on research and experience from other areas of medicine. In fact, I believe that many other chronic recurrent symptoms besides seizures respond to similar methods of control described in this book. These include headaches, asthma attacks, flare-ups of high blood pressure, recurrent low back pain, and insomnia.

Dr. Hans Selye pioneered our understanding of the human stress reaction. Faced with a real or perceived threat, the human body responds with increased activity of the autonomic nervous system. That's why acute stress produces a rapid heart rate, increased blood pressure, and sweaty palms. Selye also determined that *chronic stress* leads to prolonged periods of overactivity of the autonomic nervous system, which in turn can cause illness.

Acute and chronic stress aggravate epilepsy, causing an increase in the frequency of seizures. It might interest you to know that stress aggravates other common medical conditions, as well. For example, heart researcher Dr. Robert Eliot summarizes his findings as follows: "The evidence suggests that unresolved emotional stress pursues metabolic and physiologic pathways. . . . When acute stress such as emotional shock is superimposed upon a chronic setting of vigilance, biobehavioral factors often become important triggering mechanisms . . . understanding and measuring the impact of life-style, behavior and stress is integral to understanding and ultimately preventing acquired cardiovascular diseases."[3]

Dr. Bernard Lown shared the 1985 Nobel Peace Prize for leading International Physicians for the Prevention of Nuclear War. Previously, as a cardiologist he led a team who studied the relationship between psychological triggers and life-threatening cardiac disturbances. They found that 25 out of 117 patients had psychological triggers that precipitated their life-threatening heart irregularities. Lown concluded, "Three sets of conditions . . . contribute to the occurrence of malignant ventricular arrhythmias in a sizable subset of patients. Foremost is the presence of a psychological state intense enough to pervade and burden daily life. Most frequently it is caused by an affective depression or a sense of psychological entrapment without perceived exit. And the third is the psychological triggering event. These three factors are dynamically interrelated."[4] In other words, as poets have known for centuries, your emotions affect the workings of your heart.

Other examples support the role of stress in aggravating what appear to be strictly physical health problems. Thirty years ago, Dr. M. Friedman found that when accountants were under increased occupational stress at tax time, their serum cholesterol increased without any change in their diets.[5] Dr. Dean Ornish and his associates have collected research data indicating that a behavioral approach, similar to the approach to epilepsy described in this book, can halt and begin to reverse coronary artery disease.[6] People whose arteries in their heart are clogged may be able to open up their arteries by changing the ways they respond to other people and the world around them. Researchers at major university centers have developed ways to teach people to reduce stress and improve daily life-coping skills as a means of diminishing the disease-producing effect of the HIV-1 virus that causes AIDS.[7]

You may still be skeptical about the new concepts described in this book. Should you discuss these methods with your doctor, who might not be receptive? Indeed, many physicians and patients feel that this approach is too far out to achieve good results. Dr. Walter Cannon, the American physiologist who fathered our understanding of the physiologic basis of emotion, would not be surprised by this skepticism. Dr. James Lynch quotes Dr. Cannon as predicting in 1929, "No matter how clear and how overwhelming the physiologic evidence about the influence of emotions on the body might be, there would be deep resistance toward incorporating it into medical practice."[8]

I wish John Donne's poetic assertion that "no man is an island" could be incorporated into the current practice of western medicine, including neurology. Instead, each discipline has become its own island. There is so little communication between islands that we rarely form a chain of understanding. The mind has been split from the body; the emotions from the mind; and the soul or spirit has been excluded altogether. This book attempts to bring diverse aspects of medical and psychological knowledge together to help people with epilepsy. The intention is not to provide a viewpoint that contradicts the standard medical approach. Instead, we offer a wider viewpoint with additional tools to help you control seizures and improve the quality of your life.

As enthusiastic as I feel about the methods of seizure control described in this book, I'm painfully aware of the limitations of our understanding of epilepsy. Neurology is still ignorant of the biological causes of most forms of epilepsy. We need more effective antiepileptic drugs, with fewer side effects and fewer risks to developing fetuses. More must be learned about the positive aspects of epilepsy that foster a muse as grand as Dostoyevski's or Flaubert's, and a brush as magnificent as Van Gogh's. Finally, we must gain a greater understanding of the subtle effects of brain surgery for the control of epilepsy. Are there qualities of the individual that are cut out of the brain by the same knife that attempts to control seizures? Before taking such a risk, why don't we neurologists give more patients the opportunity to try the approach described in this book?

The "quest for a 'new neurology,' a holistic science of the person-with-the illness, rather than the mechanistic and fragmented neurology of the illness itself" is the quotation which appears at the beginning of this book. This quest is not only for a new neurology but for a new medicine as well. I believe that the people with epilepsy, like those I have introduced in this chapter and like many of you I've never met, validate this quest. You are the pioneers—the determined individuals whose personal quest for seizure control and quality of life will help to transform modern medicine.

In your notebook:

- What experiences have you had in your own life where you were able to overcome an obstacle? It doesn't matter how big or how small that obstacle was. Make note of what it was, how you did it, and how you felt afterward.
- What quality in yourself did you call on when surmounting this obstacle?

PART THREE

SEEING YOURSELF IN A NEW WAY

7

The Whole Person

One must treat the whole person.

—Wilder Penfield, M.D.[1]

Donna Andrews, Deborah Lee, and several others whom Dr. Joel Reiter has presented in the previous chapter are dramatic examples of individuals who surmounted the gravest difficulties. They saw themselves, perhaps consciously, perhaps not, as whole persons, larger than the problems they faced and able to bring what was undamaged to bear on what was. They couldn't change their history. Those events that gave rise to epilepsy had taken place, but they could think differently about that history.

It is essential in any chronic long-term illness or health problem to see yourself as a person-with-an-illness. This stance is not simply a psychological one or a stoical one of ignoring pain and disability. It has health-giving neurophysiological effects as well. Physicians routinely predict death within a few days or weeks for people with the most life threatening of diseases, and yet some of them live—or at least hang on—for much longer. Although some research has been done on the characteristics of those who appear "hardier" than others, hardiness does not explain everything. Each of us is a whole organism, not only a diseased part, and it is this wholeness that we can draw on and count on as we address the difficult questions of epilepsy.

That our attitude toward our own health affects our general well-being as well as specific symptoms is not a new idea. The first book that I read on the interrelationship between our minds and bodies was *Getting Well Again* by

Carl Simonton, M.D. and Stephanie Simonton.[2] Just as cancer was coming out of the closet, the Simontons' book and the workshops they conducted around the country for cancer patients offered a possible reprieve from the death sentence that cancer meant at the time. In *The Relaxation Response*,[3] published in the mid-1970s, Herbert Benson, M.D. reported that certain breathing and meditational practices advocated by Maharishi Mahesh and Transcendental Meditation helped to reduce blood pressure and improve circulation for heart patients. In the 1980s, the focus of this kind of mind/body research has been on the immune system and is known in medicine as psychoneuroimmunology. There is considerable evidence that stress and its consequent physical and psychological tensions depress the immune system's functioning, making illness and disease more likely.

Acknowledging that a person's mind-set affects illness or wellness is difficult for biomedical practitioners to accept. Nonetheless, departments of behavioral medicine have sprung up in medical schools around the country, and doctors trained in family medicine try to take a broader, more biopsychosocial, approach. Puzzling over my symptoms one day, my primary physician said to me, "You aren't your lab tests. They only tell part of the story."

Each of us has a range of functioning from optimum to minimum with occasional peaks of experience exceeding our usual performance and occasional bursts of negativity or worse. We need to work toward keeping ourselves at the upward end of this mental and physical scale. As Dr. Sacks states in *The Man Who Mistook His Wife for a Hat*, "A disease is never a mere loss or excess—there is always a reaction, on the part of the affected individual, to restore, to replace, to compensate for and preserve [his or her] identity."[4] We need to make sure that what we do in response to epilepsy is positive and ensures our wholeness in the best possible way.

Seeing yourself as a whole person in a positive way may not be easy to do. Epilepsy can play havoc with your life. Depending on what kind of seizures you have, they may have enormous consequences in every area of living and functioning. School, jobs, professions, personal relationships, sexuality, and family and community participation may be adversely affected. In some cases it is difficult to see what avenue other than being a victim is open to a person who is seriously damaged or afflicted with seizures. Nonetheless, at the deepest level epilepsy involves choice. Do I see myself as victimized or challenged? Do I act at the bottom of my personal scale or toward the top?

WHY ME?

Any and every illness carries meaning for our lives. Many people with epilepsy feel punished, even cursed, although they probably would not go as far as the seventeenth-century French philosopher/mathematician, Blaise Pascal. In his "Prayer to Ask of God the Proper Use of Sickness,"[5] he saw his illnesses and afflictions as punishment for his sins. But when any illness or affliction is severe enough to make a more or less normal life difficult to impossible, we begin to wonder, why me? What did I do to deserve this? Toward the end of his long prayer Pascal realizes the unknowable-ness of what he seeks, writing, "I know not which is the better or the worse of anything; I know not which is the more profitable to me, health or sickness."[6] How we think about illness, disorder, or disease makes an enormous difference. Although we cannot know what "the proper use of sickness" is in God's eyes with any certainty, we can see it in our own eyes and lives as positive and make it profitable.

THE VALUE OF PSYCHOTHERAPY

Psychotherapy can play a facilitating role in seeing yourself as a whole person. In the view of the neurosurgeon Wilder Penfield:

> Psychotherapy . . . is an essential part of the treatment of every patient with epileptic attacks. One must treat the whole person. Most clinicians are convinced that the frequency and severity of attacks can be influenced favorably when emotional problems are properly handled.[7]

I heartily agree with Dr. Penfield for a number of reasons. For one, with a skillful therapist the emphasis can be shifted from illness to wellness. "Bring out your remembered wellness," the cardiologist Herbert Benson said one day to a Mind/Body workshop at the New England Deaconess Hospital in Boston. When Donna Andrews suddenly thought, "If the damage is there all the time, why aren't the seizures?" she was making the subtle shift to the side of wellness. When you have a disabling or disordering long-term condition, remembering your wellness and able functioning may require some help. The shift is likely to be made little step by little step.

A therapist can be a real help in putting seizures into a larger and broader perspective. One day a psychiatrist said to me, "It's only a seizure." *Only* a seizure? I was shocked, then angered, thinking that he disparaged a seizure, but that was not his meaning. "Only a seizure" entailed the ability to see a seizure without conditioning it as good or bad, positive or negative, without coloring the episode with my thoughts about it. From our discussion I learned how much I still clung to my identity as an epileptic and what it would mean to let go of it. Seeing a seizure as unconditioned makes it much easier to place within a larger and more positive perspective on your life.

Another reason why psychotherapy should be an accepted part of treatment is the need to address the depression that so commonly accompanies epilepsy. There are a number of reasons for this depression. The social and psychological stresses that a person with seizures lives with are enough, in many cases, to cause depression. Recently some research attention has been directed toward identifying the psychosocial stresses. Teenagers are particularly affected because their entrance into adult life may be seriously compromised.

What is more, the medications taken to control seizures can cause or exacerbate depression. Phenobarbital is now recognized as the worst offender, but phenytoin (Dilantin) and other drugs may also contribute to depression. I took both phenobarbital and Dilantin for years, struggling a great part of the time with longer and longer periods of depression. I thought all the while that I just felt sorry for myself, that my life wasn't that bad—and indeed it wasn't.

But depression and epilepsy are more deeply linked than the stress of living with seizures or the effects of medication. Recently this relationship has been submitted to research and scrutiny. In 1986, the neurologists M. F. Mendez, J. L. Cummings, and Dr. Frank Benson[8] reported three studies that suggest deeper ties. In one study a group of people with epilepsy was compared with a group of physically disabled individuals: paraplegics and others. It was found that "depression was almost twice as prevalent" among those with epilepsy. "Suicide attempts were four times as frequent." In the second study, "All epileptics admitted in one month to a Veterans Administration neuropsychiatric hospital" were interviewed, and "80 percent of them were given an admission diagnosis of depression." The third study of almost one hundred individuals being considered for brain surgery showed that "58 percent gave a history of significant depressive episodes." Certain areas of the brain—the temporal lobes, the hypothalamus, and the amygdala deep in the brain—as well as the endocrine system are involved. There is even evidence, Dr. Frank Benson reports, that the sudden termination of seizures has brought on major depression. It seems clear that epilepsy and depression have intimate neurological links.

It is very difficult to pull yourself out of a depression on your own, especially if you have endured a number of depressive episodes. Depression takes on a life of its own over time, and it can recur more and more frequently. Frequent recurrence is called *rapid cycling*, and the sequence becomes more and more difficult to break. In addition to its neurological and biochemical elements, the personal content of a depression may be difficult to address alone. A skilled psychotherapist, whether a psychiatrist (an M.D.), a clinical psychologist, or a social worker, can help enormously in bringing out your personal experiences and staying with you while you work through them and learn to let them go or find their positive aspects.

Many seizures do not have demonstrable cause in brain injury or abnormality. When this is the case, personal history needs to be taken into account, and psychiatrists and therapists become essential. Child sexual abuse, particularly incest by alcoholic fathers and father-surrogates, is implicated in both absence seizures and complex partial seizures. In summarizing the cases he studied, Meir Gross, M.D., concluded, "For every adolescent girl who is presented to the clinician because of hysterical seizures [without organic cause], a detailed history [should] be taken that will include information about the family dynamics, with particular attention to the possibility of incest."[9] Physical abuse may cause the same symptoms in boys. These are obviously cases for both medical and psychosocial therapies.

ADDRESSING THE AURA IN THERAPY

Where a seizure begins with an aura, the series of preliminary sensations or images, the specific content of the aura may hold personal meaning. It can be addressed like the images of a dream. Experiencing fear to the point of terror or a sense of pending evil is typical. Although the fear may be aroused because certain areas of the temporal lobe and limbic system are involved, how that fear is expressed will be as personal as a dream image. When one young man was asked what his aura of fear made him think of, he said, that his mother used to tell him as a kid, "You'll burn for that," and his father used to chant, "That the devil exists there is no doubt, but does he want in or does he want out?" The burden of childhood fear, sin, and guilt still weighing on this man was suddenly apparent to him for the first time. A therapist can help a person address this kind of guilt and release it, at least to some extent.

I have found the images that preceded my own massive seizure particularly rich and rewarding. One morning, a gray-skied Sunday in late October, I was sitting on the living room couch, feeling normal enough, when suddenly I found myself staring at a book lying open on the coffee table in front of me. The book began to grow larger until the rectangular pages were folio size. At the same time the markings on each page grew larger and larger. Those on the left-hand page retained their orderliness, but those on the right began to tumble and rearrange themselves, dissolving into fiery lines and molten shapes that moved faster and faster, always growing larger and larger until I could see only the right-hand page. When it was so large I no longer saw its edges, I cried out, "I'm afraid!" I turned my head to the right, cried out, and lost consciousness completely.

Afterward I addressed those images as if they were the images of a dream. That a book was the focus of my aura seemed reasonable enough. I am a writer, and the coffee table was littered with books and rectangular magazines and sections of the Sunday paper. The disordered tumbling images on the right-hand page seemed reasonable as well. The injury that is believed to be the cause of my seizures lies in my left temporal lobe, and the left hemisphere controls the right side of the body. That the growing disorder was projected on the right-hand page made good neurological sense.

What did not occur to me until I read the psychologist C. G. Jung and the neurosurgeon Wilder Penfield was a meaning for the rectangular shape itself. This image of order, of wholeness, seemed to appear just as the wholeness of the organism, its neuropsychophysiological integrity, was about to disintegrate. Because these images of wholeness occurred early in the seizure, it seemed to me later that a return to wholeness after the disintegrating experience must be the work of consciousness. I needed to address these images and make them part of my life to achieve some degree of self-healing. In the twelve years since this experience I have not had another massive daytime seizure. I do not know if addressing the seizure's images caused that kind of seizure to go away. They may not be related, but looking at a seizure for its value seems to defuse some of its automatic power.

Intense fear is a common experience, either as an element in the aura or as anticipation of a seizure's onset. Sometimes there seems to be personal reasons for feeling afraid as in the case of the young man I mentioned earlier. More often the fear is a kind of cosmic one of losing control, of losing the known order, as it is in our fear of death. This cosmic fear seems to strike both the person having the seizure and the onlookers alike. The case of the Chicago White Sox baseball player who had a seizure at batting practice illustrates the point. His teammates panicked and sat on him to prevent the seizure from taking its course. By doing this they unwittingly mimicked a shaman's helpers who may sit on his chest to prevent a sick person's evil spirit from staying in the shaman's body.

Addressing fear in both personal and larger terms can help enormously. A certain relaxation will occur. The writer Norman Cousins once told the *Christian Science Monitor,* "Fear of disease is one of the greatest intensifying factors in that disease—and so if we don't meet that fear, we're impairing the treatment."[11] As you learn to see epilepsy in a positive light, you release yourself from fear in a very real way.

What kind of therapist is best able to help with epilepsy? I am tempted to say, a good one. Today there is a bewildering array of types of psychotherapy. Traditional verbal psychotherapy has been useful for me, particularly since I tend to be a verbal type of person. People who experience powerful internal images and dreamlike sequences during seizures may find a therapist such as a Jungian analyst or someone trained in psychosynthesis to be more helpful. In both these disciplines, dreams and imagery figure prominently. Other therapies are more physical than verbal and may be particularly appropriate, for example, the Alexander technique, bioenergetics, or dance and movement therapy. These therapies teach you to release tensions that are deeply held in your body. One Alexander teacher told me that he learned to quiet his own Jacksonian epilepsy, the trembling of one arm that had been with him since birth, with the methods he now teaches.

It is extremely difficult, however, to find a psychiatrist or psychotherapist who knows much about epilepsy. When I was first diagnosed in 1947, the two disciplines of neurology and psychiatry were practiced by the same person in the model of Sigmund Freud. In the years since then, the two specialties have grown apart, and communication between them has become poor to nonexistent. Neurology carries great prestige in the medical profession whereas psychiatry has little. People with epilepsy are poorly served as a consequence. Fortunately, a reconciliation seems possible. At the 1988 convention of the American Psychiatric Association a panel of distinguished neurologists presented a program on "Psychiatric Aspects of Epilepsy" to a packed hall.

In recent years anticonvulsant medications have been used more and more in the treatment of psychiatric disorders such as depression, manic-depression, and schizophrenia. There is a borderland between epilepsy and mental illness where seizures, often called pseudoseizures because they lack an organic basis, occur. Emotional and behavioral problems may appear alongside genuinely epileptic seizures, that is, those with an organic basis in brain lesions. The reunion of psychiatry and neurology will be all to the benefit of people with seizures from whatever cause.

Psychological factors in epilepsy have been known for over a century. The overlap between epilepsy and migraine, depression, and other mental illness was described by the great neurologist Sir William Gowers in his book *The Borderland of Epilepsy*. Published in 1907, it is now out of print, but Oliver Sacks's *Migraine*[12] draws extensively on Gowers in discussing this "borderland" between the psychiatric aspects and the neurology of epilepsy.

One evening at a meeting of an epilepsy group the chairman went into a seizure. At first he seemed to be simply listening to the discussion. Then it was obvious that his breathing had become very shallow and his eyes were vacant, unfocused. I tried to bring his attention outward by calling out to him, but it was to no avail. He twisted to the left and stiffened. The men helped him to the floor so that he would not hurt himself or hit his head. He twisted and turned back and forth and then lay still. We tucked a jacket under his head and laid another over him for warmth and went back to our meeting. Perhaps ten minutes later, his fingers grasped the edge of the table, then the top of his tousled head appeared and he eased himself into his chair. "You okay?" the man next to him asked. He nodded and we went on with the meeting. We treated this episode as just a seizure, no more and no less. It had come and gone, leaving a whole person behind.

In your notebook:

- "Remember your wellness." Make note of those systems in your brain and the rest of your body that are working well: heart, lungs, digestion, colon, muscles, vision, memory, decision making, and others.
- Describe a day or period of time, perhaps briefer or longer, when you felt you functioned at your optimum level. Don't compare yourself with others. Look only at yourself.
- Do you feel that epilepsy is some kind of punishment? If so, for what? Write about your feelings at length if you can. Think of your seizures as a challenge. What would this challenge mean in your own terms?
- Do you have sensations of fear with your seizures? Describe an episode.
- Do you have images or sensations or experiences of any kind in the preliminary moments of a seizure? Write these down. What meanings do you associate with these images?
- Make note of episodes of depression, if any, or other psychological problems. Would a psychotherapist be helpful?
- If so, search out the names of several therapists representing different methodologies and interview each before choosing one. Which one seems to make the best sense to you? Write down your reasons. Which one do you like best? Whom do you think you can work with best? A patient-therapist relationship is a personal matter. A therapist who is just right for a friend may be all wrong for you. Trust your instincts on this.

8

Understanding Strange Experiences

The air was filled with a big noise and I tried to move. I felt the heaven was going down upon the earth and that it had engulfed me. I have really touched God. He came into me myself, yes God exists. I cried, and I don't remember anything else. You all, healthy people . . . can't imagine the happiness which we epileptics feel during the second before our fit. . . . I don't know if this felicity lasts for seconds, hours or months, but believe me, for all the joys that life may bring, I would not exchange this one.

—Feodor Dostoyevski[1]

Strange experiences are so common in epilepsy that they are recognized in neurology and given names or descriptive terms. Dr. Joel Reiter has addressed the principal categories in chapter 3 and given each a thorough treatment. The living experience of these seizures can be pleasant and pleasurable, and it can be terrifying and completely disorienting. You may have the strong impression not so much that you are going crazy but that you have already gone. Because your seizures are so strange you are much more likely to take yourself to a psychiatrist than to a neurologist. There is so little awareness in the medical profession that these experiences may have a basis in the neurology of epilepsy that misdiagnoses are common, and individuals stay in therapy for years or spend long periods in psychiatric hospitals in an effort to understand and control what they think are psychological problems.

The problem of diagnosis is complicated by the fact that none of these experiences is the exclusive property of epilepsy. Everyone is subject to occasional bouts of irrational fear. Everyone is depressed from time to time. And everyone, I would guess, has had the experience of being in a familiar place and suddenly finding it unfamiliar, or of hearing something that you have never heard before but have the strong feeling that you have. You may have met someone for the first time but have the feeling that you know the person well. It is the kind of experience that leads people to think that they have in past lives lived in this place or with this person. In the terms of epilepsy, as Joel Reiter has explained, these are called déjà vu (seen before) and jamais vu (never seen).

These are just examples on the extensive list of strange experiences that people with epilepsy may experience. Some are more disorienting and problematical than others. They are the most difficult and troublesome—and also potentially enriching—to the persons who go through them. In this chapter we will consider what strange experiences mean to your life and whether the medications you take for seizure control may be eliminating experiences you could find valuable or even enjoyable. A psychotherapist with a knowledge of epilepsy can help you consider this dilemma. The self-care methods in Parts IV and V are particularly important if you choose to go without medication or with minimum medication in order not to lose these experiences.

In his insightful book, *The Man Who Mistook His Wife for a Hat*, the neurologist Oliver Sacks describes an elderly woman patient whose seizures took the form of involuntary memory. Before her seizures, which were caused by a stroke, she had never been able to remember the least detail of the first five years of her life. Her seizures seemed to unlock this stored memory and became for her a source of great satisfaction. She saw her seizures and the stroke "as health, as *healing*." [Emphasis Dr. Sacks.] "Such cases are exciting and precious," Dr. Sacks comments, "for they serve as a bridge between the physical and the personal, and they will point, if we let them, to the neurology of the future, a neurology of living experience."[2]

A lovely teenager told me one day in a counseling session of her experience with déjà vu. Her spells had set in when she was seven or eight, striking most frequently in school. Although they would be followed by a severe headache, her mother tended to discount them until they became more frequent in high school. A well-informed neurologist was able to diagnose this déjà vu as simple partial seizure and prescribed phenobarbital. The medication left her continually fatigued, the spells were not entirely controlled, and at sixteen or seventeen this young woman took the courageous step of going without medication, allowing the episodes to occur and take on meaning in her life.

Religious experiences of a highly personal nature are commonly reported by persons with epilepsy. Does this mean that religious experiences are nothing but the pathology of wildly firing neurons in a certain part of the brain? Here the material premises of biomedicine fall short. I heard a psychiatrist tell a deeply religious woman, "Spirit is not a medical concept." In my workshops a notable number of participants have a well-developed religious life of an experiential nature. Once medication controls the seizures, these mystical experiences may be greatly lessened or vanish completely. Here again you need to ask yourself what such experiences mean in your life. Do you want to lose them?

Some New Testament scholars believe that St. Paul had epilepsy and that his conversion experience on the road to Damascus was a seizure. There are other incidents scattered through his letters that suggest seizures. The Swiss psychologist C. G. Jung saw them as psychological in origin and "erroneously explained as epileptic. The fits were a sudden return of the old Saul-complex which had been split off by his conversion just as the Christ-complex was before."[3] St. Paul's case is an excellent example of that borderland of confusion between the neurological and the psychiatric. If Paul had seen a neurologist or a psychiatrist rather than the Christian disciple Ananias on the street called Straight, the history of the western world might be quite different.

The neurologist David Bear cites Moses and the revelation of the commandments, and Mohammed and his tour of heaven that takes place in the few moments a pitcher of milk is spilled, as indicative of seizures.[4] The visions of Ezekiel[5] strike me as very seizure-like because they happen without warning. Once the initial visions with their elaborate imagery of thrones, chariots, and wheels had occurred, the others are introduced abruptly: "The word of the Lord came to me" or "In the eleventh year, in the third month, on the first day of the month, the word of the Lord came to me." My own experiences of visionary states begin and end with the same abruptness. In one extraordinary vision, Ezekiel received the detailed architectural specifications for the new temple in Jerusalem, a creative vision if there ever was one.

I also think it is highly likely that St. Teresa of Ávila had epilepsy. She was subject to "fainting fits" as an adolescent, and she suffered a four-day coma in her mid-twenties. When she had returned to the convent near Ávila and recovered to a degree, she began to have the "raptures," visions and visitations that continued throughout her life. She herself found them "not like [the experience] of fainting or convulsion; in the latter nothing is understood inwardly or outwardly," but she describes her experience in epilepsy-like terms:

> He takes away the breath so that, even though the other senses last a little longer, a person cannot speak at all . . . and the hands and the body grow cold so that the person doesn't seem to have any life, nor sometimes is it known whether he is breathing. This situation lasts but a short while. . . . But . . . the will remains so absorbed and the intellect so withdrawn, for a day and even days.[6]

She writes of "another kind of rapture—I call it flight of the spirit"[7] when the "spirit is carried off," often leaving the body. This kind of experience occurs frequently in epilepsy. It is also shared by some shamans in tribal societies who journey to the spirit world to apprehend causes of illness or misfortune. A common neurological basis may underlie these experiences.

When the great Russian writer, Dostoyevski, experienced moments of oneness with the godhead just before he lost consciousness, he described them in his notebooks and letters. There are a number of characters with epilepsy scattered through his work, but Prince Myshkin in *The Idiot* has the seizures that most closely resemble Dostoyevski's own ecstatic states. These obviously enriched his life and work.

Other kinds of psychic experience are also common. A young woman with epilepsy described her experience of extrasensory perception to a medical audience in Boston. Her seizures began after a serious automobile accident, and with them came the ability to read other people's thoughts. Her neurologist urged her to test her powers of ESP, and she went to the dog track where she was able consistently to predict the winners. Once her medication controlled the seizures, she lost this uncanny ESP.

Her case is a reminder that the oracle at Delphi in ancient Greece was often selected from women with epilepsy and that the prophesying epileptics in late antiquity and the Middle Ages held special status. There is probably a neurological basis for their ability to predict events and read unspoken thoughts.

In his initial Edinburgh lecture, "Religion and Neurology," later published in *The Varieties of Religious Experience*, the great American doctor/psychologist/philosopher William James commented, "Even more perhaps than other kinds of genius, religious leaders have been subject to abnormal psychical visitations. . . . Often they have led a discordant inner life, and had melancholy [depression] during a part of their career. They have known no measure, been liable to obsessions and fixed ideas; and frequently they have fallen into trances, heard voices, seen visions, and presented all sorts of peculiarities which are ordinarily classed as pathological. Often, moreover, these pathological features in their career have helped to give them their religious authority and influence."[8] The neurophysiological conditions that underlie these experiences may well be the same as or similar to those that produce epileptic seizures.

Epilepsy is often diagnosed in or attributed to persons who excel in artistic, literary, or even sociopolitical realms.

Vincent van Gogh was diagnosed with epilepsy during his lifetime, a condition probably exacerbated by his drinking of absinthe and the absorption of toxic chemicals. The paints that gave the bright colors he loved were heavy with lead and chromium, metals now known to affect the nervous system. His bursts of rage and demanding friendships characterize what behavioral neurologists today call an *interictal* personality, one with certain characteristics such as emotionality, lowered sexual drive, religiosity, and obsession exhibited between seizures.

A *musicogenic* seizure, one where the person hears music during the aura or one that is triggered by music, is common in epilepsy. The composer Hector Berlioz described his own seizure-like experience as he listened to another composer's music:

> My whole being seems to vibrate. . . . The emotions . . . produce, little by little, a strange agitation on the circulation of the blood; my pulse beats violently; tears which usually give evidence of the crisis of a paroxysm, indicate only a progressive stage and greater agitation and excitement to follow. When the crisis is really reached there occur spasmodic contractions of the muscles, a trembling in all the limbs, a total numbness of feet and hands, a partial paralysis of the nerves of vision and hearing.[9]

The precision of this astonishing account displays Berlioz' medical as well as his musical training. The passion and intensity of his description bring to mind the passion and intensity of his great work, *The Damnation of Faust*.

The list of writers who had or are believed to have had epilepsy is long. Not only Dostoyevski but Flaubert, Lewis Carroll, Edward Lear, Molière, Petrarch, and Jonathan Swift are prominent. The writers are equaled by great religious leaders like Swedenborg and the others already noted, and political leaders like Alexander the Great, Julius Caesar, Napoleon, and Peter the Great. The American black leader, Harriet Tubman, was struck in the head by an overseer, and afterward suffered hour-long lapses of consciousness. The insights that she brought out of these periods are believed to have guided her in her work as a leader of the underground railroad, bringing some three hundred slaves north to freedom.

The persistence of "the firm belief in the occurrence of epilepsy among the most adventurous conquerors . . . religious reformers . . . and some writers, artists and scientists" led the eminent Otto Kanner, M.D., to write in 1930,

> It would be a fascinating study . . . to try to establish the connections between the epileptic attack and its aura on one hand and the world conquerors and reformers with their attempts to reach out into the cosmic vastness on the other.[10]

Recently behavioral neurologists have attempted just such studies. Unfortunately, their conclusions tend to be pejorative of the experiences, identifying them as hypergraphia, moralistic excesses, and religiosity. It is ironic that the medical entity called epilepsy, which is often experienced by the most intuitive patients, is the province of the least intuitive and most intellectual specialty in medicine today. In 1902, William James commented, "Medical materialism then thinks that the spiritual authority of all [religious] personages is successfully undermined . . . by the dependence of mental states on bodily conditions."[11] He adds, "Scientific theories are organically conditioned just as much as religious emotions are."[12]

Few of us would dare to think of ourselves in the same breath with these intellectual and creative giants. Our experiences are not likely to change the world, but they may have great meaning for our personal lives. If they are lost through medication, you may want to ask yourself whether the gain in seizure control outweighs the loss in experience. The meaning of this loss should also be a consideration in evaluating candidates for surgery, as Dr. Joel Reiter has suggested in chapter 4.

Much more difficult to see in a positive light are the problems of memory involved in epilepsy. Loss of memory and mental confusion often follow a massive seizure. I have had as much as five days of some memory loss and considerable fogginess following a seizure, and they are commonly experienced by others. There isn't much to do but take care of yourself and wait till they pass. Most often complete memory is restored, although you may not believe it the first time you experience memory loss.

In another variety of epilepsy a period of amnesia called a *fugue* occurs. One young woman told a seizures workshop group that she would be in the kitchen and the next thing she knew she would find herself in the living room, not knowing how she got there. Many people have this kind of experience, but it is likely to occur more frequently when it is related to a seizure condition. A fugue state, however, can be much more extensive than the preceding example. People are known to buy plane tickets and arrive in strange places not knowing who they are or where they came from, while others may commit minor offenses like petty theft in a state of amnesia. One neurologist told me of a vegetarian who shoplifted several packets of meat from a supermarket without any memory of doing so. This example may be another one, like St. Paul, of a cutoff complex breaking through.

A massive seizure on a public street is embarrassing enough, but other forms of epilepsy can be even more distressing because they are not recognized as seizures. Automatic behavior, uncontrollable speech, and highly emotional public responses are hard to cast in a positive light. A college teacher told me, "I simply tell my classes the first day that if I go to the light switch and turn it on and off, it's a form of epilepsy, and it will be over in a minute or two. I'd prefer not to have to do it, but a couple of kids have come up to me and said it made them feel better about some hidden problem that they had." One young woman's seizures began in early adolescence and took the form of her crying out, "Wait a minute! Wait! Wait!" Medication did not help, and she suffered through a traumatic adolescence. As a young adult she has found that she tolerates some medication much better. Her work with a psychiatrist on the meaning of waiting at that early point in her life has helped to reduce the number of her seizures. In addition, she has discovered the benefits of reducing stress and restricting exacerbating substances.

Highly emotional public responses are particularly embarrassing for men who are supposed to be tough. They are often not a seizure but may be a consequence of being prone to seizures. Being able to brush off the incident with a certain nonchalance is possible for outgoing persons. Simply letting it happen and going on is another alternative. These kinds of incidents are always more noticeable to you than to others.

Perhaps the most disturbing episodes of all are those of having visions, hearing voices, or having extended spontaneous reveries. These can be creative and enhancing, but they are often negative or even suicidal. You may be left shaken and confused. The voices may deliver ultimatums or instructions that raise the question of whether they should be followed. Because these experiences carry an authority, as if from a power outside yourself, they can be deeply disturbing.

I am often asked in my workshops what to do about the instructions delivered by vision or voices or in extended reveries. If you are frightened and worried, you should report the episodes to your neurologist. Some change in medication may eliminate these episodes entirely. If you find them disturbing but interesting and perhaps of value to your life, then you can address them in a variety of ways. A psychotherapist who is fluent in dream imagery and symbols will be immensely helpful.

First, ask yourself if the instructions indicate a course of action that in the cool light of reason you want to take. Then, look at the instructions not so much literally as metaphorically. For example, if you feel suicidal during an extended reverie, ask yourself if there is something in your life you want to be free of. Treat suicide as a metaphor, not as an imperative. A woman painter told me that voices had instructed her to give up painting because it put her in competition with her sister, who was also a painter. To give up her art, she felt, would break her heart. With a therapist she addressed her sense of competition with her sister and in the process turned their relationship into a highly creative and mutually stimulating one. Her fear and anxiety were dispelled, and the episodes of hearing voices disappeared. Often the voices, reveries, or visions speak of deeply held fears, and once these have been addressed, release into a fuller life is possible.

Not every voice speaks from fear and negativity. In one epilepsy workshop a middle-aged man said that he had been given instructions on how to control his seizures in a dream, but he couldn't remember them afterward. If he had remembered the instructions, he would need to examine them objectively and rationally for their value, not follow them blindly just because they had been given.

Curious bodily sensations are also frequent occurrences. During her first seizure, a middle-aged woman had an out-of-body experience much like the one St. Teresa of Ávila described. This woman's experience, however, was not of a religious nature. She seemed to hover in the upper corner of the room and saw herself at work in the room below. Similar but less extreme is the sensation that an arm or a leg doesn't belong to you. This kind of bodily experience can be addressed both as epilepsy and as indicative of your possible inner psychological state.

Premonitions of future events, telepathic communications, and extrasensory perception, although not exclusively epileptic, are common experiences for persons with seizures. Again you need to ask yourself what these faculties mean to you. Some people value them highly. They are the source of the faculties used by a trance-medium or spirit-diviner, and in other cultures they are trained and cultivated. What you do about them depends very much on how disturbing or interesting you find them. With the current interest in channeling, psychic readings, and healing, there are numerous workshops in psychic abilities offered around the country. Although I have had a number of experiences of this kind, I do not consider myself particularly psychic, but I have taken some psychic training because of my deep interest in epileptic experience. In its early stages at least, psychic training teaches you to be consciously aware of the sensory cues we pick up from other people without knowing it. More advanced training, however, goes beyond the sensory. For example, telepathy has very little to do with immediate sensory perception. Here intuition and unusually deeply felt connections are involved. Experiences of this kind go beyond the boundaries that our society has set. If you wish to cultivate these powers, you need to consider seriously what this may mean to your life and to your personal relationships.

The psychiatrist Stanislav Grof and Christina Grof have described many similar experiences as a crisis of spiritual emergence. Dr. Grof writes:

> Transpersonal crisis . . . is characterized by a striking accumulation of instances of extrasensory perception (ESP) and other parapsychological manifestations. In acute episodes of such a crisis, the individual can be literally flooded by extraordinary paranormal experiences. Among these are various forms of out-of-the-body phenomena.[13]

A real danger here, Dr. Grof emphasizes, is in seeing yourself as chosen and endowed with messianic purpose.

Behavioral neurologists tend to reduce these experiences to their neurological basis in the temporal lobes and the limbic areas of the brain. Initially they called such experiences psychomotor and temporal lobe epilepsy and now call them complex partial seizures. Because these seizures lie in the borderland between epilepsy and mental illness they are now being called temporal limbic syndrome or TLS. It is difficult for people trained in scientific, materialist modern medicine to deal positively with these varieties of epileptic experience.

My own view is to value the experience, to treat it as a dream for its symbolic and metaphorical meaning and possible personal direction, and divest it of fear and anxiety. Often when this kind of experience is addressed, it does not recur.

In conversation with a psychotherapist friend one day, I told him of a strange but pleasant and amusing psychic experience of my own. He has never had a seizure, but he had had a similar experience, and he commented, "Don't try to analyze it. Don't try to figure out what it means. It just happened, and that's kind of wonderful." In this instance I took his advice.

Although the strange experiences discussed here are commonly part of certain types of seizures, they are not exclusively the province of epilepsy. Other people have them, too, even though they do not have seizures. They do not prove that you are crazy, nor are they necessarily undesirable events, even though they are beyond our society's usual boundaries. An appropriate openness to and examination of these experiences can lead to a real enhancement of your self-concept. You may be able to discover and alleviate deeply entrenched fears that have limited your growth and mental outlook.

In your notebook:

- Describe any strange or curious experiences you may have had: religious, psychic, intuitive, sensations of dissociation from your body or out-of-body experience, and others.
- What do these experiences mean to you?
- In what ways do these experiences enrich or disturb your life? You may wish to discuss these experiences with your neurologist or psychotherapist. Write down your reasons for or against doing so.

9

Seeing Yourself in a Larger Context

*N. N. from Argos, epileptic. This man during his sleep in
the curative chamber saw a vision: He dreamed that the
god [Asklepios] approached him and pressed his ring . . .
upon his mouth, nostrils, and ears—and he recovered.*

—Fragment from the healing center at
Epidaurus, Greece, third century B.C.[1]

Because of the secrecy that has surrounded epilepsy, and the consequent lack of support and understanding from the world around us, most of us feel or have felt isolated and alone in our affliction. This sense is greatly relieved when we see ourselves in the context of epilepsy's long and fascinating history. All the questions of epilepsy have been addressed again and again in every age, in every culture, in every healing system, everywhere in the world. What is it? What causes it? How can it be treated? Each historic period, each culture and its medicine, have interpreted epileptic seizures according to the particular premises and assumptions of that time and place. Epilepsy like all other diseases and disorders occurred and still occurs within the context of a culture, and the culture colors not only the medical approach but the way we experience it as well.

The records of epilepsy are as old as the written history of the world. Not only is it mentioned in the earliest written texts and tablets of western culture but other cultures of the world have addressed it in their own ways. Epilepsy occurs

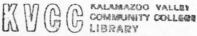 KALAMAZOO VALLEY
COMMUNITY COLLEGE
LIBRARY

all over the world, and it is not confined to certain historic times or places, by climate or geography, or by age or race, as are many diseases. Probably because of its dramatic nature, it was impossible to ignore and was subject to many interpretations. The Greeks called these strange episodes *epilepsy*, meaning "to be seized by a god or demon," and the word has stuck ever since.

EPILEPSY IN ANTIQUITY

The earliest reference to epilepsy is on a scrap of tablet dating from 2000 B.C. found in the Persian Gulf region. A few centuries later Article 278 of the Code of Hammurabi specifies that anyone who buys a slave who has a seizure within one month of purchase can return the slave. This practice, incidentally, is also recorded in Egypt, about the third or fourth century A.D., and was also the practice of American slave holders less than two hundred years ago.

More important for western medicine are the treatises on health and healing brought together under the name of one fifth-century Greek healer, Hippocrates. In his great text "On the Sacred Disease" Hippocrates addresses epilepsy's dual nature as a physical phenomenon and as divine or demonic possession. Much of this tract heaps scorn on those who regarded epilepsy as demonic possession.

> It appears to me to be nowise more divine nor more sacred than other diseases, but has a natural cause from which it originates like other affections. Men regard its nature and cause as divine from ignorance and wonder, because it is not at all like to other diseases.[2]

"Neither truly do I count it a worthy opinion," he wrote farther on, "to hold that the body of man is polluted by god, the most impure by the most holy."[3]

In spite of Hippocrates' eloquence, epilepsy as demonic possession was the order of his day and persisted. Treatment in ancient Greece followed methods used at the Asklepion at Epidaurus, the greatest healing center of its day. After

N. N. from Argos made the journey to the Asklepion, he underwent rites and purifications, took herbal emetics and physics, preparing for his night in the curative chamber. When he was considered ready, he slept in this sacred place that was half below ground, and there he dreamed of Asklepios, the presiding god of the healing center and the god of both patients and physicians. Asklepios pressed his ring against N. N.'s mouth, nostrils, and ears, three openings where evil might enter. The ring itself is remarkable. Greek gods, to my knowledge, did not wear rings. The ring seemed to arise as a spontaneous dream image of wholeness. It seems almost redundant to add, "and he recovered."

The circle or ring as a common image in an epileptic seizure was noted by the Swiss psychologist C. G. Jung. When the great Canadian neurosurgeon, Wilder Penfield, probed the brain of his epileptic patient during surgery, conscious and able to speak, she had a vision of a circle in a square. A "circular image of this kind," Jung commented, "compensates the disorder and confusion . . . through the construction of a central point to which everything is related. . . . This is evidently an *attempt at self-healing*" (his emphasis).⁴ The ring's appearance in N. N.'s dream seems to corroborate Jung's and Penfield's twentieth-century research.

In ancient Greece two gods were singled out as the particular gods of epilepsy. Pan and Hecate were both associated with fertility rites far more ancient than the Olympian gods, and as they were adopted into the Olympian family, they continued to carry an association with a darker, more instinctual side of human nature. Pan was known for the terrifying suddenness of his appearances. His name is the root of our word panic, and suggests the swiftness of an epileptic attack as well as the fear that may go with it. Hecate was absorbed into the Olympic pantheon as one of the goddesses of the underworld, the one most feared and most closely associated with evil. She had many forms and often appeared as dog-headed or with three savage dogs, suggesting the wild, untamed instincts of her earlier form as a fertility goddess of Thrace.

It is not difficult to imagine how Hecate came to be associated with epilepsy. The fear and anxiety many people feel in the early stages of a seizure often intensify as an apprehension of evil. When N. N. from Argos, in the fragment that graces this chapter, dreamed of the god's ring, it was pressed against the three openings in the body through which evil was believed to enter. One man in his mid-thirties tells me that his massive seizures frequently begin with the sense of an evil presence, that he will wake in the night knowing something evil is out there, beyond his bedroom door, where he can hear it or him—he uses both pronouns. He is so terrified that the hair rises on the back of his head and the back of his hands. He tries to tell himself that there is nothing and nobody out there, but he must get up and look and then lock his bedroom door before he can fall asleep again. He had never had such an experience before the accident that caused his seizures.

To the onlooker an epileptic episode is very strange. The sudden loss of control over physical movement, the loss of consciousness, the swiftness of its coming and going, suggest something supernatural or death itself. Hippocrates noted a seizure's resemblance to death throes, the unconsciousness, the thrashing, and often the foaming at the mouth. A woman once described her brief seizures to me as "many little deaths." A common seizure experience is of leaving the body and watching oneself, very much like the near-death experiences reported widely today.

The appearance and the symbolism of death and return to life are unmistakable in epilepsy. The ancients recognized it and both honored and feared it. Hecate was, as we have seen, a fearsome deity of death and the underworld. Among the Romans, who had many names for epilepsy, there were two, morbus daemoniacus (demonic disease) and morbus deificus (god-like disease), that express these mixed feelings. Today we can see the motif of death and renewal not only in the seizure itself but in the depression, a kind of death to life, that often accompanies it. Again I am reminded of the high incidence of suicide and suicidal gestures among people with epilepsy.

EPILEPSY IN THE CHRISTIAN ERA

Although in antiquity epilepsy was seen as both morbus daemoniacus and morbus deificus, and both views persisted into Christian times, the emphasis shifted to epilepsy as demonic possession.

When the father brought his epileptic son to Jesus to be cured, it is clear that the boy was possessed by an "unclean spirit." In the Gospel According to Mark 9:14 (and following), the father speaks to Jesus, saying:

> "Teacher, I brought my son to you for he has a dumb spirit, and wherever it seizes him, it dashes him down and he foams and grinds his teeth and becomes rigid." . . . And they brought the boy to [Jesus]; and when the spirit saw him, immediately it convulsed the boy, and he fell to the ground and rolled about, foaming at the mouth. And Jesus asked the father, "How long has he had this?" And he said, "From childhood. And it has often cast him into the fire, and into the water, to destroy him; but if you can do anything, have pity on us and help us." And Jesus said to him, "If you can! All things are possible to him who believes." . . . Jesus rebuked the unclean spirit, saying to it, "You dumb and deaf spirit, I command you, come out of him and never enter him again." And after crying out and convulsing him terribly, it came out, and the boy was like a corpse, so that most of [the crowd] said, "He is dead." But Jesus took him by the hand and lifted him up, and he arose.[5]

The vivid description of a grand mal seizure leaves no doubt that this is epilepsy. The belief that it was caused by an unclean spirit and cured only by Jesus' enormous powers to exorcise it is apparent. Is this account credible to us today? The answer is yes. That seizures can vanish abruptly is one of the unexplained phenomena of epilepsy. Being treated publicly by the greatest healer/teacher of the day would have had a profound psychological effect on the boy.

The view that epilepsy is evil persisted in the following centuries. During the Middle Ages, the Church Fathers concerned themselves with epilepsy as possession. There are long passages in Latin that record their opinions supporting their belief that still has vestiges today. In an interview with the *Atlantic*,[6] the former California Congressman Tony Coelho said he had been refused entry into the Jesuit religious order because of his seizures. It had been the Order of Jesus' practice since its founding in 1540 to deny admission to anyone with epilepsy.

In the Middle Ages and later allegorical meaning was assigned to epilepsy. It was analogous to the sin of pride and suggests the well-known adage, "Pride goeth before a fall."

In 1640 when Governor John Winthrop led some 800 Puritans to the Massachusetts Bay Colony, he brought these instructions with him:

> For ye falling Sicknesse Purge first with ye Extract of Hellebore (:black hellebore I meane:) and instead of St John's Wort, use pentaphyllon, (or meadow Cinquefoile:) use it as aboue is said of St Johns Wort, & God Willing he shall be perfectly cured in short or longer tyme, according as the disease hath taken roote.[7]

Although Governor Winthrop's instructions sound practical and unemotional, within sixty years the seizure-like "fits" of a ten-year-old girl, Elizabeth Parris, would set off the witch trials in Salem that concluded in nineteen men and women being put to death.

At the same time, in seventeenth-century Europe, the science of medicine was growing and diverging from the practice of religion. Sir Thomas Willis, an English physician and researcher, published his *Anatomy of the Brain and Nerves*[8] in 1664. It was the first book to reveal the nervous system, and it was illustrated by the great architect-to-be Christopher Wren. The circumstances in which a person with epilepsy lived, however, were hardly improved by this great work. In seventeenth-century Britain, one-third of the occupants of the madhouse at Bedlam were persons with seizures. Living conditions in the asylum were unspeakable.

They were hardly better in the eighteenth-century French women's prison LaSalpêtrière in Paris. There the mad, the epileptic, the unwanted, and the unmarriageable were confined for life along with prostitutes and petty thieves. Around 1860, a young neurologist named Jean Charcot became the director of LaSalpêtrière and began to make the observations that separated epilepsy from insanity and criminality. A young Viennese neurologist, Sigmund Freud, came to LaSalpêtrière to study under Charcot. Epilepsy, like mental illnesses, was being described, rationalized, and given its own scientific classification as a neurological disorder. Some forms of epilepsy have been well served, but others, those now called partial seizures and complex partial seizures or TLS (temporal limbic syndrome) still defy classification as the province of neurology or psychiatry.

Hanging on the wall of Jean Charcot's examining room was a portrait of John Hughlings Jackson, perhaps the greatest neurologist of his day and certainly the greatest to work in the field of epilepsy. He described one form of seizure that carries his name to this day: Jacksonian epilepsy. The era of heroic medicine based in scientific research and minute clinical observation and dominated by medical personalities had dawned.

Treatment during the nineteenth century was usually bromide of potassium. Although it worked in high dosages, it had serious side effects. One doctor commented as he showed his fourteen-year-old patient to other doctors, "As you see, he is broken down in appearance, has large abscesses in his neck, and is altogther in a bad condition. But this is better than to have epilepsy."[9] The alternatives, of being tossed into the asylum at Bedlam or perhaps castrated, were indeed worse than a few abscesses. What shows through the doctor's remarks is the persistence of the belief that epilepsy was a bad or evil condition.

The residue of these beliefs continues today and is expressed in social, economic, and legal stigma. When I was first told in my early twenties that I had epilepsy, I knew instantly that I must never tell anyone. The fear of being ostracized was almost instinctual. Not long ago I was making a presentation on seizure interventions to the staff of a center for retarded adults. Afterward, one of the staff took me aside to tell me about his own case, first making me promise not to mention it to anyone for fear that he would lose his job. The fear that society will punish us for this affliction is so persistent that I have come to feel it is closely bound to the experience of the seizure itself. Both the person who has the seizure and society believe at a deep level that a seizure means to be taken over by some irresistible evil force.

Today, as a religious view has declined and a scientific view dominates, epilepsy is seen not so much as an evil but as a negative, something that should be wiped out. It may affect learning in school, or keep you from getting a driver's license or a good job. It is no longer considered a disease. It rarely progresses—but it can be disabling.

At the same time the belief in epilepsy as morbus deificus also persists. David Bear, M.D.,[10] has recently raised the question of whether epilepsy or its underlying neurological conditions is not an indicator of the potential for high creativity in many fields. He suggests that epilepsy may indicate the basis for "transcendant artistic production" and transformational visionary states. To have such suggestions coming from a distinguished researcher in the neurology of epilepsy is indicative of a potential shift in biomedical thinking.

EPILEPSY IN OTHER CULTURES

Nonwestern healing systems have addressed the phenomenon of epilepsy within their own cultural contexts. The traditional medicine of China is based historically on The Yellow Emperor's Manual of Internal Medicine. Roughly the equivalent of the Hippocratic treatises, the volume was written in about 300 B.C., but is believed to record practices from much earlier centuries. Traditional Chinese healing sees all disease as a consequence of an imbalance between the yin and yang forces of the universe. The ill person is brought back to health by treatments from an elaborate and elegant pharmacopia of herbs and roots, powders of bones and minerals, and through acupuncture and massage. The objective is to bring that person into proper relationship with the universal vital force, chi, and to permit this force to flow smoothly through the body. In traditional Chinese medicine epilepsy is seen within this context.

In Ayurvedic medicine, the traditional medicine of Hindu India, the body and other forms of matter are considered the densest forms of spirit and not separate from it as in western medicine and science. (My educated guide through the Elephanta Caves near Bombay kept referring to "the living rock.") From this viewpoint, epilepsy may be seen as an uncontrolled expression of spiritual energy. Practitioners of Kundalini Yoga such as the late guru Muktananda and Gopi Krishna had experiences that strongly resemble convulsive seizures. Practitioners of Kundalini work to control and channel these expressions of spiritual energy. Hatha yoga, the physical exercises widely practiced in the West, is a healing system where each pose or asana helps to relieve certain symptoms. Certain asanas such as the shoulder stand series and "the pose of tranquility" are considered especially beneficial to the nervous and circulatory systems.

The traditional healing systems of many tribal societies have found ways to treat the individual with seizures. In Zimbabwe, when it was still Rhodesia, the physician, Michael Gelfand, talked with five nganga, traditional healers, about their treatment of epilepsy. All of them believed it was caused by a disturbed or angry ancestor spirit or by the curse of a sorcerer or witch. All disease was explained on this basis, and an ancestor spirit was believed to be much easier to deal with than a sorcerer's curse. Once the seized person was revived with inhalants, he would be treated with purgatives or enemas, body washings, and incisions. Then, either the disturbed ancestor spirit or the witch would be addressed and released from the person through an elaborate ritual. One nganga described the treatment ritual to Dr. Gelfand:

First the powder of the mutovic root is mixed with castor oil. This is burnt and the patient inhales the fumes with his head covered by a sheet. Then the mapfufu powder is mixed with oil and smeared over the whole body which is then wrapped in a bag. . . . The head is covered with an old blanket and the patient is pushed into an antbear hole. He is then pulled out of the bag which is left in the hole. Some of the mapfufu mixture and dry grass are set alight in the hole. When the patient leaves the spot, he must not look back.[11]

This description is striking. The symbolic death, burial, and rebirth are obvious. In addition, fire plays a part, cleansing and destroying the past. For the cure to be effective the person must go into a new life—"he must not look back"— thoroughly cleansed of the old, thinking of himself and seeing himself in a new way.

A somewhat different approach is taken by the traditional healers of the Yoruba in Nigeria. They also believe that all illness is caused by a disturbed ancestor spirit or some kind of black magic. To determine which is the cause they use a method of divination called *ifa.* When ifa does not indicate either cause, then it is assumed that the person with epilepsy has been called by the gods to become a trance-medium. The trance-medium functions in that society by going into an altered state of consciousness to answer questions brought to him or her by ill or perplexed individuals.

Where the Yoruba culture has been transplanted to the New World, the same view is held. In Brazil, one psychiatrist is said to train his patients with epilepsy to become trance-mediums, achieving seizure control in some 80 percent. In the Cuban healing system, *santeria*, seizures may indicate a potential santero. Where the Cuban has melded with the Puerto Rican *espiritismo*, the same belief is held. To become a healer, however, the person must learn to control his seizures. The possibility that seizures may be faked in order to qualify for a prestigious calling is also recognized.

In his book, *Lightning Bird*, the British scientist Lyall Watson writes:

> In Africa the epileptic myth . . . sees the symptoms as evidence
> of supernatural possession. Anyone who has such a seizure is
> regarded . . . as blessed by the spirits. . . . And the epileptic,
> far from being a social outcast, [has] a special place in
> society.[12]

Nothing is done, he states, to stop a seizure. This remarkable
little book is about one white man, Adrian Boshier, who had
a massive seizure while visiting a Northern Lusotho tribe.
Afterward Boshier was invited to take training as a spirit-
diviner (similar if not identical to a trance-medium). He did
so, and for two years he was seizure-free. What accounts for
such a period of control in terms of western neurology no
one seems to know. Having seizures go away and then return
is not uncommon. However, something different may have
been involved with Adrian Boshier. Making positive use of
the neurological conditions that make for uncanny ESP and
a highly intuitive personality might account for this period
of remission.

Among the traditional Navajo, seizures have three causes.
One is incest, another frenzy witchcraft, and a third, the
potential to be a hand-trembler. A hand-trembler is a trance-
medium who diagnoses illnesses and prescribes the appropriate ceremonial for healing. The ceremonies for epilepsy
differ according to the causes of the seizures.

In his book, *Shamanism*, Mircea Eliade[13] reports that
seizures, particularly when they begin in adolescence, are
indicative of a potential shaman, a priest-healer. In most
tribal societies, however, epilepsy is believed to indicate
latent powers of a lesser kind such as a trance-medium or
spirit-diviner.

Treatment in most of these societies involves using re-
gionally available potions and herbs, often massage, and
then healing ceremonies that may involve a large part of the
community. These healing rituals are methods of symbolic
healing that address the whole person and attempt to restore
her to a right relationship with the gods and ancestors, with
forces of the universe, and with human society.

Many western students of symbolic healing believe that

it is a valid system in its own right. It has its own premises, obviously different from western medicine, but rational ones nonetheless. Although healing rituals in other societies strike us as bizarre, every healing system invokes powerful cultural symbols. Think of our associations with the white coat, the framed diploma, and the mysterious technologies that penetrate the body. To a certain extent, doctors act like priests as they mediate between us and esoteric knowledge. Most of us feel better after we have seen our doctor, whether he has prescribed medication or not. Whether we call this feeling the "placebo effect" or "awakening the inner healer," or use the great missionary doctor Albert Schweitzer's metaphor of the doctor within each patient to explain it, the result is a healing effect on the whole organism.

That other healing systems are effective should come as no great surprise. All healing systems help people to feel well and to get well. Nevertheless, we tend to believe that only western biomedicine, our system, really works. To test this conviction Arthur Kleinman, M.D.,[14] conducted a study comparing Taiwanese patients treated by western medicine and those treated by traditional methods. He found that the numbers cured by each were within a few percentage points of each other. The efficacy of traditional healing was sustained in follow-up studies a year later.

Seeing ourselves in historical and cross-cultural contexts helps us to view our own case histories in a new way. Taking a long perspective over centuries not only reveals epilepsy's rich and fascinating history but also shows how views of epilepsy have changed. Becoming aware of this historical framework led me to realize that there is nothing immutable about our contemporary interpretation of epilepsy. It, too, will change. Epileptic symptoms are universal, but interpretations of them differ according to what Arthur Kleinman calls the "explanatory model" of different societies. Biomedicine restricts itself to neurophysiological explanations whereas other cultures regard as critical the individual's relationship with cosmic, societal, and supernatural forces. Neither explanatory model is wrong, and both relieve symptoms and sometimes effect cures. When we see epilepsy in the context of other cultures, we change our own perspective. The limits imposed on us by our own society can be seen for what they are—only one way to view epilepsy's symptoms. This realization frees us and makes us more whole.

At this moment in time we find ourselves at a turning point. Our biomedical concepts of wellness and healing are expanding to include processes and methods that encourage an individual's wholeness, that validate personal experiences, and that broaden our view of epilepsy. When we adopt practices to bring out our "remembered wellness," release our deepest fears, and see ourselves as part of a rich and varied historical experience, we move into a new and different life.

We are on the threshold of a new way of seeing. As the nganga of Zimbabwe instructed, "Do not look back!"

In your notebook:

- Write down the ways your epilepsy is received in the mini-culture of your family, relatives, friends, and religious community.
- How do you believe epilepsy is seen in the larger world around you?
- How are you affected by these attitudes?
- Be sure to leave space to add to your written notes as more comes to mind a day, a week, a month from now.

PART FOUR

OBSERVING YOURSELF

10

Noticing Circumstances and Conditions

I woke up one morning . . . and found myself lying on the floor, up in the stalls of the cathedral . . . lying in a pool of blood, having bled profusely from the nose, which no doubt had received a heavy blow in my fall . . . and had been lying there exactly an hour . . . and I remained kneeling when the others left the building. . . . So I had the place all to myself, to sleep off the attack (epileptic, no doubt), . . . Luckily I met no one on my way back to my rooms, for I was a pretty figure! With my face and shirtfront all covered with blood. My doctor found me to be out of health generally—at least the digestion was out of order— and this may have caused the attack. Anyhow, the result has been a great deal of headache, and unfitness for brainwork. . . . You laugh at me for the "fearful agonies" you say I suffer "over a coming sermon," but I really think sermons may have something to do with it . . . preparing them takes a good deal out of me . . . I have been "taking it easy," now, for a good while, and my headaches are getting fewer, and my brain recovering its usual power.

—Lewis Carroll[1]

In one remarkable letter the author of *Alice's Adventures in Wonderland* describes vividly his epileptic seizure and gives us a model for self-observation. He tells us what happened. He notices the circumstances and conditions surrounding what happened and suggests what may have triggered the seizure. He reports his doctor's comments and his progress in recuperation.

Lewis Carroll expresses himself in such contemporary terms that he might have written his letter last week. Not only does he observe his physical condition when consciousness returns but he realizes that he has no memory of how he got into the cathedral. The massiveness of his grand mal seizure would have overpowered the brain. His immediate reaction is one of shame. He hides from the others as they leave the early morning service. This spontaneous feeling of shame is familiar to most of us who have seizures. Even the Greek physician, Hippocrates, noted this impulse in his fourth-century B.C. treatise on epilepsy. It takes Lewis Carroll a while to recover from the seizure, and then he manages to get back to his rooms without being seen. When he consults his doctor, the doctor finds his health not up to his usual functioning, particularly the digestive tract. Constipation perhaps? And he is under what we would call "stress" as he prepares one of his brilliant sermons. His headache, which often follows a seizure, persists, and so does the mental confusion that will pass after a few days so that his remarkable intellect will recover "its usual power."

These are the points you need to remember as you learn to observe yourself and take notice of the circumstances and conditions in which your seizures occur. Each of us is different. You can learn from Lewis Carroll and others, but you must observe yourself carefully to determine which conditions and circumstances trigger a seizure for you.

The conditions and circumstances that set up your internal preconditions for a seizure can be emotional or psychological in origin, physiological or environmental, or a combination of two or more of the above. You need to observe and reflect on your own particular case.

Dr. Joel Reiter and epilepsy counselor Donna Andrews recommend keeping not only a seizure log to record the occurrence and severity of seizures but also keeping a journal with entries that describe in careful detail what happened and why you think it happened at the particular time that it did. Since the neurological preconditions for a seizure—for example, epileptiform electrical patterns or a damaged area in the brain or a possible genetic predisposition—may be present all the time, the specific conditions when a seizure breaks through are particularly important to recognize. Once you know what they are, you can do something about them. Robert Efron, the neurologist whose patient stopped her seizures with the smell of jasmine, urges self-observation as the single most important facet of treatment for epilepsy.

You may want to consult a psychotherapist to help you clarify and work through volatile psychological and emotional issues that are difficult to sort out by yourself. For example, many people tell me of their sense of a rising tide of unreasonable fears like the ones we have discussed earlier. The very act of consciously observing such interior feelings is a significant step toward dispelling them. At one point I stopped and asked myself why I felt such fear and panic when I knew I was perfectly safe, and it may have been the first step in dispelling that fear. The presence of a skilled counselor can help us reach the detachment we need as we observe disturbing or strong feelings about our inner experience.

General conditions of health and effects of life-style also influence the conditions conducive to seizures. You may need to consult your primary physician about some exacerbating problem. Your nutrition and dietary habits may not be ones that improve your functioning. Here an assessment by a nutritionist may be helpful. Unless you keep a daily log of what you are really eating, and the amount you are consuming, you are not likely to know exactly what you are taking in and what it may be doing to you—and not doing for you.

Probably the single most common cause for a seizure to break through is forgetting to take your prescribed medication. To be effective, anticonvulsants must be maintained at certain levels in the bloodstream. Thus, they must be taken at regular intervals throughout the day and blood must be checked for the therapeutic level of the medication. Sometimes other medications interfere with the effectiveness of anticonvulsants. For example, vitamin B_6 can interfere with the efficacy of Dilantin.

Physical tension is something I have observed in many participants in my seizure workshops. It seems to be a general condition for persons with epilepsy. Physical tension means tight, often rigid muscles that restrict movement and circulation. The neck and shoulders are particularly susceptible. I first noticed this tension as I worked with retarded adults who have seizures. Then I began to notice it in myself. Not only were my movement and circulation impaired but my breathing was restricted because of the tight chest. Often in stressful circumstances my breathing was so shallow that it seemed almost to have stopped. Once I realized that I was subject to extreme tension, I was able to release it and not let it accumulate.

One of the two grand mal seizures I have had in the past twenty years was a nocturnal attack. It occurred after a strenuous week where every day left me tense and exhausted. I was under extreme stress and at the same time overexposed to heat and sun. Every night I had a glass of wine with dinner. I was in circumstances where I had no time or space to take care of myself, to pay attention to my diet or do relaxation exercises. When I awoke the next morning to headache and vomiting, my usual pattern, I knew what had happened. I returned home and consulted my neurologist, and he asked, "What about alcohol?" Until that moment I had forgotten about the wine with dinner every night. I looked back in my notebook and found I had jotted down, "Drinking too much alcohol." Although a glass of wine with dinner is not considered too much necessarily for a person with epilepsy, it is for me when I have one night after night. What other people with seizures can do without ill effects is not possible for me. Altogether this nocturnal seizure was a revealing experience. Out of it I learned what circumstances and conditions can trigger a massive seizure for me.

The importance of noticing the conditions and circumstances under which a seizure occurs can't be overemphasized. Once they are known, the external circumstances and conditions can be altered. The internal conditions can be changed to some extent as well.

It is fascinating to see that the shame Lewis Carroll felt immediately following the seizure has passed by the time he writes to his aunt. Now he is speaking of his seizure openly and without reticence. As we observe our experiences and the circumstances and conditions that surround them, and then relate them to someone important to us, we are already making a significant step toward greater well-ness.

Every time a seizure breaks through, ask yourself these questions:

Are you remembering your medication at the prescribed times?
Do you feel tension and rigidity in your body?
What were you doing that may have overtaxed your system?
Were you under emotional stress?
What were the reasons for the stress? Did it arise from problems at work? A difficult personal relationship? Placing unreasonable demands on yourself?
Were you under physical stress? From fatigue? Alcohol? Illness? Menstruation? Too much sun or exposure? Dehydration? Weight-loss diet? Excess fluids? Competitive workouts? An excessively sedentary life? Constipation?
Were your diet and nutrition out of balance?
Had you changed any part of your life in recent days?
Were you particularly affected by something that happened in the world around you?

Think of yourself as Lewis Carroll as he wrote his letter to his aunt, and notice everything that you can about your conditions and circumstances.

In your notebook:

- Ask yourself the questions listed above and record your experience.
- Which condition or conditions are the most pertinent for you? Describe these in detail. If you have trouble writing, follow the outline of Lewis Carroll's letter: what happened, what the doctor found (if you consulted one), what your activities were leading up to the episode.
- Had you taken your medication at regular intervals, if you are on medication? Were you taking any other medications or health aids? Ask your physician if any temporary drug may have interfered with the effectiveness of your seizure medication. Write all this down, including your doctor's responses.

11

Recognizing Warning
Signals

He had warning of the attacks, but he had to to be sure of
the arrangements, and to know that he could have the
privacy he need[ed].

—Vivian Noakes, *Edward Lear*[1]

Recognizing your aura, the warning signals that
precede a seizure, is of critical importance in being able to
do something about the seizure. Not every variety of epileptic episode begins with these premonitions, but they are
common for many people with seizures. The Greek physician Galen gave them the name of *aura*, a Greek word
meaning "breeze," in the first century A.D. Today medical
terminology calls them *prodroma*, another Greek word
meaning "running before." You need to experience a series
of seizures with an aura in order to recognize it.

A massive seizure can obliterate the memory of an aura.
If Lewis Carroll had a warning signal, either he did not
recognize it because he had not had previous seizures or he
lost the memory of it in the severity of the attack. Edward
Lear, the mid-nineteenth-century author of *The Owl and the*
Pussycat, recognized his aura and had sufficient warning to
take himself to a safe hiding place. One woman member of
a seizures workshop said that she knows a seizure is coming
when she notices that she is slurring her words. "When I
start to twitch a little," a young woman told a group, "then
I know it's coming."

Some people are not conscious of their own auras but
depend on others to recognize them. One participant in an

epilepsy workshop said that he couldn't observe his aura, but his wife said that she could. She found him irritable and erratic in behavior before the onset of a seizure. For some, their aura is so subtle that only after a careful educating process can anyone detect it.

What does the aura consist of? Many different feelings, sensations, and activities occur because different areas of the brain are involved. You may already recognize the premonitory experience in your own seizure pattern.

Your aura may be an entirely internal experience. For the woman who sniffed jasmine, Dr. Efron's exemplary patient, the aura was a smell that did not exist in the outer world. Queasy sensations in the stomach may be predictive. Voices, sounds, inner music, and images that have their life within the brain may be the prodroma for some people. Dramatic mood swings from amiability to rage and possible violence may indicate the stirrings of a seizure. You may feel "spacey" and light-headed or simply nervous and jumpy. Surges of sensation may rise up the back of your neck into your head, or your whole body may tingle. Your powers of intuition may dramatically increase. You are the only one who can observe these indicators before they reach the point of overt acts.

The fear that has been discussed in previous chapters is a common experience before a seizure. A man of thirty told me that terrifying waves of fear began to rise in him one day as he took care of an antique shop for a friend. He was terrified that he would break some valuable antiques and that he would have a seizure in public. As the fear intensified, he managed to lock the shop, go out on the street and hail a taxi, hang on through the ride to his apartment, pay the driver, and get up the front walk and inside the building before he fell unconscious to the entrance hall floor.

There are other types of aura that only an observer will be able to see. Some persons move a part of the body in a certain way, lifting an arm, turning the head. Often the eyes lose their focus and the pupils dilate. My husband tells me that I would always call out his name in a tone of voice I never used at any other time. At one time I was working with an autistic man who had seizures, and no one had been able to detect any indicators of a seizure coming on. He could not communicate any internal sensations he might have felt. After being with him through one or two seizures, I realized that his face always began to turn blue just as the seizure began.

The importance of knowing the signs of an aura is enormous. Like Edward Lear and the young man in the antique shop, you may have time between the onset of the aura and onset of the seizure to take yourself to a safe and private place. The need for safety is obvious, but the need for privacy is almost as important. Hippocrates, that acute observer, noticed this need twenty-four centuries ago:

> But such persons as are habituated to the disease know before-hand when they are about to be seized and flee from men; if their own home be at hand, they run home, but if not, to a deserted place, where as few persons as possible will see them falling.[2]

There is another important reason for being able to recognize your aura. Recognition makes it possible to stop the seizure from going full course. There are almost as many ways to stop a seizure as there are auras. Again it is a highly individual matter. How to use the aura in stopping a seizure is discussed fully in Part VI.

Sometimes it is difficult to tell when the aura ends and the seizure begins. Fear, anger, and rage may be one or the other or both. Automatic behavior may occur as aura or as seizure. Certain physical indicators—the skin turning blue or the eyes losing their focus—are very close to the seizure itself. You and an observer may need training to recognize onset and be able to act quickly.

In your notebook:

- Do you experience an aura? Describe it. Does it occur close to the seizure or is there a certain amount of time between its onset and the seizure?
- Does another person notice that you do or say something or appear different habitually before a seizure sets in? Describe this behavior.

PART FIVE

PREVENTING SEIZURES

12

Finding Ways to Change Your World

Purpose comes to [the brain] from outside its own mechanism. This suggests that the mind must have a supply of energy available to it for independent action.

—Wilder Penfield, M.D.[1]

The sense of being a whole person gives each one of us a feeling of strength. Being able to observe our own condition and describe it enhances that feeling. Knowledge and information about epilepsy, what it is, how and why it is treated in certain ways now and in the past, strengthens us further. Now comes the time to act on that feeling of strength, to take independent action by asking yourself, What can I do to help my brain and body control these seizures?

Of greatest importance is to have a supportive environment. You may have it already, which is a great asset. If you do not, there are a number of resources that can provide considerable support.

We live in an age when epilepsy has come out of the closet, and every one with seizures is indebted to the demystifying effect of modern medicine for this openness. None of us needs to live as Edward Lear did in the nineteenth century, never daring to tell anyone of his affliction and never daring to marry or have intimate relationships for fear of its discovery.

Personal acceptance, however, is often very difficult. Individuals in particular family settings often need help in

131

developing that family as a support system. Social workers, counselors, and psychotherapists can be enormously helpful here. In the counseling I have done, I find two areas of special concern: the family's acceptance of a member with seizures and the support needed for particular interventions. Any one using self-care initiatives is greatly in need of support from others who understand and approve of what you are trying to do.

Immediate families tend to be either overly protective or angry and rejecting, often both, and neither position is particularly helpful to the person with epilepsy. From time to time you need protection, to be shielded from public exposure and to be prevented from injuring yourself, but in between these times it is far better to be treated like any other member of your family or group. Epilepsy's unpredictability is a strain on everyone, however, and certain types of seizures—odd or uncontrollable behavior, fits of rage—may strain other people's tolerance to the breaking point. You will need to realize yourself what those around you may be enduring, and in their turn they need to see your needs for varying amounts of protection and help. Sharing this book with your intimate circle will encourage a larger and deeper understanding of the epileptic experience.

You also need to be willing to relinquish any special status that epilepsy has given you, no matter if it is the status of victim or of special privilege. This does not mean that you should throw yourself into activities that are inappropriate for you. It means that you accept the present conditions of your life as simply the conditions of your life.

Where some condition exists that is beyond your power to change, it may be necessary to find another home. An abusive or alcoholic parent or other family member is one such condition. Another is an isolating living arrangement. With American mass transit in general disarray outside major cities, being unable to drive can be difficult. Today, however, many communities offer transportation for the handicapped, the homebound, and the elderly, with regular trips to shopping malls, entertainment, and churches. One young man told me of his living arrangements in a shared house where his room was the old sun porch with a Spanish tile roof. Since his seizures could be stimulated by certain sounds, he dreaded the nights of rain beating on the tile roof. Eventually he persuaded one housemate to trade rooms with him, but if he had not, he would have been forced to search for another living arrangement. By making such a change, if you need to, you will be greatly reducing the amount of stress and tension you live under daily.

An informed and sympathetic companion during these strange experiences is enormously reassuring. Even though in the midst of a seizure you are unconscious of that person's presence, you will know before and afterward that you are not alone. In my seizure workshops I ask that everyone who can do so bring a support person. Then both supporter and the person with seizures have the same information and training. Deeply felt support from parents for children with seizures is especially important. There are a number of recorded cases where a parent seeing the onset of a child's seizure can do something to arrest it. Not long ago a mother told me that she stroked her son's face when he told her that a seizure was beginning and the seizure stopped. The successful use of the inventive procedures described in chapter 21 requires a support person's trained observation and quick action.

The onset of a seizure can be so frightening and disorienting that the afflicted individual forgets even those seizure-controlling methods practiced the longest and most effectively. In my own case, I practice deep diaphragmatic breathing almost every day in meditation, but when I felt one seizure begin, terror prevented me from remembering this method at first. With someone close by to remind me to relax and breathe deeply, to close my eyes and visualize my body relaxed, I could bring this technique into use immediately. When I did so, I dispelled the fear and minimized the debilitating effects of the seizure.

Not all of us have a live-in support person, however. In this circumstance support groups can help enormously, and they provide additional social acceptance for those who do have a partner or supportive family.

Support groups are common these days. There are support groups for single parents, for widows, for the divorced, for cancer and heart patients, for anorexia nervosa, for the parents and families of afflicted persons, for those trying to overcome addictive behavior or substances. The most famous and the one that led the way is Alcoholics Anonymous. AA is not an open discussion forum but a group that requires a commitment and imposes a twelve-step program. Most epilepsy support groups are of the open forum type, although some have a limited agenda and a limited number of meetings.

Who sponsors epilepsy support groups? The local epilepsy society or local affiliate of the Epilepsy Foundation of America may hold small group meetings. Hospitals often host numerous support groups and advertise their meetings, and some corporations sponsor special groups among their employees. At one large computer firm employees have arranged to create their own network of persons with seizures. They have programmed epilepsy on the menu and trade experiences and tips through the in-house computer system. Those with access to Internet can tap into a nationwide bank of personal experience with epilepsy.

If no group exists in your area, your neurologist or physician may be able to put you in touch with others who have epilepsy.

Since epilepsy continues to carry a burden of social stigma, the openness in a support group can be personally liberating. The exchange of experiences with others may change your perspective. "There are people who are so much worse off than I am," one man told me in commenting on the group meetings he attends. If you believe as I once did that there is only one kind of seizure—your kind—you will find the variety of epileptic patterns astonishing. In addition, everyone develops his own ways of coping, which are often helpful to others.

One drawback of support groups is that they can reinforce negative feelings of hopelessness and victimization. In a productive support group members help one another maximize their best efforts. As people with epilepsy, we can do something to help ourselves, to feel better about our lives, to help our medication work better, to reduce the number of seizures and relieve their severity, perhaps even to eliminate them. Alcoholics Anonymous urges one day at a time, one step at a time, and it is wise advice. Every time we do what we can, even a tiny step, we open up the possibility of being able to do more. Others around us who believe in us help us to take the next tiny step, to use what we have available for independent action. Even more, freeing ourselves from secrecy releases a deeply held tension.

In your notebook:

• Attend a support group meeting. Make notes of what you shared and what others expressed. What did you find most interesting? How did it help you?
• If there is no support group in your area, ask your physician if she can put you in touch by telephone with someone else with seizures. Make notes of your conversations and what you find most interesting.

In a special place in your notebook, list the following information for easy access:

Support person:
Address:
Telephone:

Support group:
Meeting place:
Meeting time:
Telephone:

Local epilepsy society:
Address:
Telephone:

Contact the following national source of information on support groups:

Epilepsy Foundation of America
4351 Garden City Drive
Suite 406
Landover, Maryland 20785
1-800-EFA-1000

13

Releasing Stress and Tension

*I really think sermons may have something to do with it,
preparing them takes a good deal out of me.*

—Lewis Carroll[1]

Long before stress became widely recognized as a
factor in many illnesses and diseases, Lewis Carroll realized
that composing a sermon as well as anticipating giving it
put him under unusual strain. It was perhaps enough of a
burden on his system to precipitate an epileptic seizure.
Today it is well known that stress produces neurophysiological changes in the body, and that these changes may
exacerbate seizures.

What is stress? It is the body's response and reaction to
changed circumstances outside and inside itself. Something
happens that we interpret as threatening. You are out for a
walk, let's say, and a huge dog barks at you. The brain
immediately sends signals through the hypothalamus and
the pituitary. Hormones are released that stimulate the adrenal gland that sits on top of the kidney. Adrenalin then
circulates in the bloodstream aided by your pounding heart.
The adrenalin stimulates the liver to release its stored blood
sugar—glycogen—that will give the body what it needs if
you have to run. At the same time circulation to the extremities and the stomach is reduced. The stomach tenses, and
breathing becomes faster and shallower. Now you discover
that the dog is tied. You don't have to run. Your body must
now handle all the residue of tensed muscles and surging

adrenalin and blood sugar that would have been burned off in a sprint to safety.

This bodily reaction of fright/flight or fight has served us well over the ages. We got away from enough predators to be here today, but we are no longer living under the circumstances in which this internal system developed. Today we are more likely to be subjected to innumerable low-level daily jolts of stress, and these take their toll in habitually tensed muscles, shallow breathing, and anxious states of mind.

Persons with epilepsy live under a triple burden of stress. First, there are the stresses of daily life that affect everyone. Second, there are the anxieties of having an unpredictable and erratically occurring symptom that is misunderstood by many people. Third, there are epilepsy's particular stressors that vary from person to person.

Some research has been devoted to the relationship between stress and seizures. Mariah Snyder, R.N., Ph.D., Dean of Research at the University of Minnesota School of Nursing, has concluded one study. Other studies confirm stress as an exacerbating factor.

Many individuals find a definite relationship between stress and tension, and seizure occurrence. One woman told me that the number of her seizures rises and falls with the amount of stress in her family life. While he held a difficult job directing a halfway house, a young man endured numerous seizures. After he resigned, he went seizure-free for months. Others find that they survive a stressful week at work only to have a seizure on Saturday morning, and still others make it to their vacation, only to have several seizures once the stress eases. A middle-aged man told a seizures workshop that he had his most dramatic seizure as a high school student just as he confronted the school bully in a face-off. In my own case, social and family tensions must interplay with other abuses—a minor amount of alcohol and dehydration and loss of sleep—before a seizure will occur.

How can we avoid stress? It is probably not possible. Life is stressful and always has been. Our bodies would not be fitted with a complex neurochemical fight-or-flight reaction if it was not. It is not stress itself that takes its toll but our inability to be aware of its effect on our body and our need to expel tensions in appropriate ways.

Out of her research on stress and seizures, Mariah Snyder[2] developed a checklist of stressors commonly experienced by her research subjects, all persons with epilepsy. Take a few minutes to read and think about these stressors. Being aware of the pressures in your life increases your ability to relieve them.

Rank   *Stressor*

_____ Need to take medications regularly
_____ Uncertainty about when a seizure will occur
_____ Increasing memory loss
_____ Unable to get driver's license
_____ Others not understanding epilepsy
_____ Lack of control over situation
_____ Limitation on type of activities
_____ Losing driver's license
_____ Frustration with medicine not working
_____ Frustration that others assume you're not competent
_____ Side effects of medications
_____ Difficulty getting insurance
_____ Unable to be "just like others"
_____ Overprotectiveness of family/friends
_____ Dependency on others
_____ Fear of injuring self
_____ Cost of medications
_____ Being restricted in use of alcohol
_____ Fear about having children as they may have epilepsy
_____ Fear about sexual activity and marriage
_____ Rejection by others
_____ Fear others will find out about your epilepsy

Add any other concerns you have to this list as you rank them in order of priority for you.

The next two chapters are devoted to ways of releasing stress and tension. Chapter 14 gives you the kinds of relaxing exercise that particularly help persons with seizures. In chapter 15 you will find ways to achieve a deeper and more penetrating state of relaxation with an emphasis on patterns of breathing. Both are of primary importance to anyone with epilepsy or with any stress-affected illness. These are the methods that help us to clear our bodies of stress and tension and to develop stress-relieving habits of movement and breathing.

In your notebook:

- What stresses are you constantly under in your own life?
- Which of the stressors in the stressor list apply to you? How do you rank them? Which two or three seem to you to be the most prominent in your life? Perhaps none of these really bothers you. Write an account of your experiences with those that affect you.
- If you have had a seizure after a stressful incident, describe both the stressor and the seizure as Lewis Carroll does in his letter.
- Reread the chapters in Part IV and think again of yourself as a person with epilepsy. Observe and make note of your between-seizure self and your wellness.
- Remind yourself daily of the following:

    The brain is essential to life.
    I want my brain to act calmly and normally.
    I will do everything I can to help my brain to act calmly and normally.

- Make note of any discussions with your psychotherapist about deeply held fears in your personal life. Expand them further in your notebook.

14

Relaxing Exercises

*The walking [Edward] Lear always enjoyed—it was the
most certain way of keeping off his attacks of epilepsy;
and the world was a happier place when he was outside
and on the move.*

—Vivian Noakes, *Edward Lear*[1]

Many of us who experience epileptic seizures feel
that our bodies betray us. That we cannot depend on our
bodies affects our total attitude toward ourselves. It exacer-
bates the sense of mind/body separation and reinforces our
mistaken belief that we have little control. Because of this
record of betrayal we may not trust ourselves sufficiently to
undertake what we need most: daily physical exercise.

The parents of children with seizures often are particularly protective and may restrict their child's activities for
fear of injury. An exception was presented in the TV series,
"The Brain." The parents of a seven-year-old boy with multiple daily absence (petit mal) seizures decided to let him
ride his bicycle in spite of his condition. His mother said,
"Better a broken leg than a broken heart, a broken spirit."
This parents' choice between two worries was a conscious
decision on behalf of the whole child.

A daily exercise program is perhaps the easiest and
simplest of self-care initiatives. It provides the greatest relaxation for the entire body and helps to eliminate the buildup
of stress and tension. What could be better for people with
seizures? Before the advent of modern medications Edward
Lear found that exercise gave him the greatest relief from his
"Terrible Demon." "Hours of sedentary life," he wrote,

141

"make me boil over—a steam force which is let off by walking, but bursts out in rage and violence if it has no natural outlet."[2]

Your exercise program should be gentle. Muscles should be flexed and stretched, not abnormally tightened. Weight lifting and other kinds of body building should be moderate. Your exercise routine should minimize competitiveness. You are not pitting yourself against anyone else, nor are you in training for the Olympics, swimming the English Channel, or trying to look like Jane Fonda or Arnold Schwarzenegger. Your program is for relaxation, muscle tone, and a sense of well-being.

Choosing the proper kind of exercise is key to improving your sense of well-being. Again, you need to observe yourself and your responses. One man who participated in a seizures workshop could not drive because of his epilepsy, and he would run the several miles to and from our meeting place. His doctor told him running was all right, but he began to observe that he felt overstrained by the long-distance run. Choosing the proper kind of exercise and regulating its strenuousness are keys to using exercise to improve your sense of well-being.

Here are some suggestions for gentle exercise.

Easy jogging or alternately jogging and walking.

Fast walking—until you are breathing hard. Swing your arms.

Bike riding over gentle terrain, with a support person.

Low-impact aerobic exercises for beginners.

Swimming, with a support person.

Yoga. These exercises stretch and strengthen the body.

Dancing—Square dancing, folk dancing, and line or round dancing (ballroom dance steps choreographed for singles). They all require concentration, movement, and rhythm, and the groups tend to be lively and relaxed.

Gentle strengthening exercises like leg lifts, deep-knee bends, sit-ups, windmills. Do what you feel you need to give yourself strength and flexibility without straining.

Exercise twenty to thirty minutes a day. An exercise class helps keep you disciplined. Not only do you have support from the other participants but you have the added incentive of having paid your money!

While you are exercising, pay attention to your body and its wonderful systems. Most of them give us unflagging support throughout a lifetime with no time off. Think of these systems: the heart and the vascular system, the lungs, the amazing way that nutrients are carried to all parts of the body and waste products are automatically removed, the digestive tract from teeth to rectum, the astonishing circuitry of the brain with its perhaps one hundred billion neurons, the entire sensorium that brings us sights, sounds, smells, tastes, and textures. Notice and be thankful for what is going right.

Give a little encouragement to those parts that need it. Rub a sore muscle. Massage a stiff knee by rubbing it between your hands so quickly that heat develops. Lie flat on the floor for a few minutes and simply sense your body, the whole works, before you ask it to get up and go.

PROGRESSIVE RELAXATION

Another effective form of relaxation exercise is called Progressive Relaxation. Mariah Snyder, R.N., Ph.D., dean in charge of research at the University of Minnesota School of Nursing, conducted a research study on its applicability to seizures. Although not a large number of persons in her study found relief, because they failed to commit themselves seriously enough to carry through on the exercises, Snyder reports that "four persons practiced [progressive] relaxation on fifteen or more days each month, and three of the four had a decrease in the number of seizures."[3] In other words, 75 percent of those who practiced regularly decreased their seizures!

The fourth person experienced a slight increase in seizure activity. This finding is important to notice, too. It illustrates the magnitude of individual and seizure differences and the necessity to observe your own response and what works for you.

Another particularly valuable point emerges from Mariah Snyder's research: Regular continuing practice is necessary for positive results. Self-help practices must be done daily, and if not daily, then almost daily and certainly with great regularity. If you don't do them, they can't work any more than anticonvulsant medication can work when not taken regularly. The benefits of self-care are not just a swallow away. You need to commit yourself to their practice. When you do, the rewards are worth the effort!

Progressive relaxation is not new. A Chicago psychiatrist, Edmund Jacobson, introduced it in the United States in 1929, and it was known in Europe before that. Today it has become a standard element in stress reduction training. Mariah Snyder writes, "Jacobson believed that tensing the muscle and then releasing the tension would help the person become aware of unnecessary muscle tension. The premise is that muscle relaxation would interrupt the stress cycle and contribute to reduction of anxiety throughout the body."[4]

Other researchers who have studied the effectiveness of progressive relaxation in reducing seizures have obtained results similar to Mariah Snyder's. In a Swedish research study of a group of adults, the median seizure reduction was 66 percent,[5] and in three American studies, "88 percent of the participants experienced some seizure reduction" with a median reduction rate of 49 percent.[6] These results are impressive and should influence anyone with epilepsy to take progressive relaxation seriously.

Stress and anxiety accompany seizures. Any relief will increase a general feeling of good health, and some people have reduced their incidence of seizures with these exercises.

A brief form of progressive relaxation is the series of exercises given below. When Joan Borysenko, Ph.D., then the head of the Mind/Body Workshops at the New England Deaconess Hospital, Boston, introduced her version of these exercises, her instructions were to do each of the exercises "in conjunction with [conscious] breathing. Tense each body part to its maximum as you breathe in. Hold as long as comfortable. Let go of tension gradually as you exhale. It's interesting to notice how easy it is to appreciate feelings of relaxation when they follow feelings of tension. Take a few breaths between tensions/relaxations, continuing to allow relaxation to develop in the part you just tensed on each successive outbreath."[7]

The exercises are:

1. Curl your toes tightly. Hold. Relax.
2. Flex the feet, bringing the toes toward the knees. Hold. Relax.
3. Tense the muscles of the calves. Hold. Relax.
4. Tense the kneecaps. Hold. Relax. Take a few breaths.
5. Tense the muscles of the thighs as if you were trying to lift your legs against a weight. Hold. Relax.
6. Tighten the buttocks, making them hard, like sitting on rocks. Hold. Relax.
7. Take a deep breath and pull the abdomen in and harden it. Relax. Take a few breaths—don't forget these.
8. Take a breath and tense the whole upper body. Hold. Relax.
9. Make fists with your hands. Hold. Relax.
10. Extend your hands back at the wrists as if bending the hand up toward the elbow. Hold. Then relax.
11. Tense the forearms. Hold. Relax.
12. Tense the upper arms. Hold. Relax. Exhale.
13. Raise your shoulders up to the ears. Be careful not to tense too hard here. Let them drop. Relax.
14. Raise your eyebrows and furrow your forehead. Hold. Relax.
15. Squeeze your eyes shut. Hold. Relax. Exhale.
16. Smile, pulling back the corners of the mouth and baring the teeth. Hold. Relax. Exhale.
17. Drop your jaw and stick out your tongue. Hold. Relax. Exhale.

18. Lift your shoulders gently toward your ears again. Hold. Relax. Exhale.

19. Pull your shoulders down, stretching the neck muscles. Hold. Relax, letting the shoulders rise to their natural position. Exhale.

These exercises are simple but extraordinarily effective for relaxing the body. It is important to tense the muscles and then relax them. The alternation makes for the effectiveness of the exercises.

STRETCHING

Simple stretches will also release tension in the body. The ones described below come from Hatha yoga, the kind of yoga that is concerned with the physical body. One of the principles of Hatha yoga is that you should exert yourself only to the point where you begin to feel uncomfortable. Just stretch to the point where you feel your limit. Each day your outside limit will change, and over a long period it will expand. I do these exercises twice a day, and I have much greater flexibility in the evening than I have in the morning. Some days I can do them more easily than on other days. It is fascinating and a kind of wonderment to notice how differently the body responds at different times.

An easy series of exercises:

1. *The tree:* Stand with your feet parallel and three to four inches apart. Stretch your arms over your head, fingers extended. Stretch upward without hunching your shoulders. Stretch and relax. Inhale as you stretch up; exhale as you relax. Repeat two or three times, slowly. Notice how you feel.

2. *The fountain:* Stand with your feet apart about the same width as your shoulders and lift your arms above your head, making a circle with your fingertips touching. Bend sideways as you exhale and let your fingertips sweep the floor or as close to it as you can come. Inhale as you swing to the other side and lift your arms to the starting position. Repeat slowly, several times beginning to the right and several times beginning to the left. Be sure to exhale as you bend and inhale as you lift.

3. *The moon poses:* This is a series of several postures.

The first: Inhale as you raise your arms level with your shoulders. Exhale as you bend to touch your left hand to your right foot. Inhale as you straighten. Exhale as you bend to touch your right hand to your left foot. Inhale as you straighten. Let your arms fall to your sides.

The second: Lift your arms above your head and clasp your fingers. Bend to the right, exhaling. Inhale as you straighten. Bend to the left, exhaling. Inhale as you straighten.

The third: Stretch upward, turning the backs of your hands together. Exhale as you lower your arms and clasp your hands behind your back. Inhale. Exhale as you bend backward. Inhale as you straighten. Exhale as you bend forward, lifting your clasped hands above your back. Inhale as you straighten. Bend to the left, exhaling and lifting your arms above your back. Bend to the right, exhaling and lifting. Inhale as you straighten. Let your arms drop to your sides and stand comfortably. Repeat five times.

RELAXING THE NECK AND SHOULDERS

Stress and tension tend to settle in the muscles of the shoulders and neck, and the neck protects perhaps the single most important passageway in the body. Arteries carrying the essential nutrients of oxygen and glucose to the brain, the spinal cord protecting nerve tissue, the throat and its passages for food and air are all contained and highly vulnerable in the neck. We all know the pain of a pinched nerve in this area, and how tension here contributes to a headache.

To keep the neck and shoulders as relaxed as possible, the following exercises[8] are notably helpful:

1. Sit forward on a straight chair. Lengthen your spine and keep your chin level. Pick out an eye-level spot on the wall opposite you. (These can be done at a desk.)

2. Turn your head from side to side, gently pressing against your limits. Repeat five or six times.

3. Let your head fall forward, your chin to your chest. As you inhale, roll your head to the right and back. As you exhale, roll your head from center back around to its original position. Repeat five times rolling left, five times rolling right.

4. Let your head fall forward, your chin to your chest. Lift your head straight back as you inhale. Exhale as your head falls forward to your chest again. Repeat five times.

5. Look straight ahead and lift your shoulders to your ears. Roll your shoulders backward, squeezing the shoulder blades together. Release and let your head fall toward your chest. Repeat five times.

6. Looking straight ahead, lift your shoulders to your ears and roll your shoulders forward and down. Exhale as your head falls forward. Repeat five times.

7. Roll your head from side to side like a pendulum, feeling the stretch and maybe hearing the crunch in your neck muscles. Repeat six or eight times.

As you do these exercises, notice how your neck and shoulders feel. Do your shoulders settle into a more comfortable and natural position afterward? Do you observe greater mobility in the movements of your head?

As I have practiced these exercises, I have greatly increased the mobility in my neck. The daily tensions that tend to settle in the neck and shoulders are released and do not accumulate day after day. The exercises help to prevent and relieve the headaches that many people with epilepsy have as well.

OPENING THE UPPER CHEST

The "chicken wing" or dry land breast stroke is another exercise to open the lungs, relax the upper chest, and increase your breathing capacity. Lift your arms shoulder high and stretched out in front of you—bend them at the elbows to make "chicken wings"—and exhale as you bring your arms or elbows forward. Inhale as your arms sweep backward like a swimmer's breast stroke. Even infants can be gently taken through this exercise as part of their daily play.

HELPING THE FEET

Foot discomfort occasionally afflicts persons with seizures. Numbness and tingling, swelling, sore big toes, or a curious sensation of wearing tingly booties can be more than a minor irritant for some people. Can anything be done to alleviate these conditions? Here are a few suggestions:

Give yourself a foot massage. Sit up in bed where you have support for your legs, lean over, and massage your feet. Press your fingertips into the balls and arches of your feet. On the insteps press your thumbs along the pathways between the bones and ligaments that connect to your toes. Squeeze along the big tendon in the back of the ankle. Spread your toes apart and flex them. Even better, ask your support person to do it for you while you lie back and relax.

Exercise your feet by standing barefoot on a rug. Rise on the toes of one foot, then the other, descending toe to heel. Do a few of these with your other exercises.

Find a way that especially helps you. When her feet are giving her great discomfort, a woman I know goes to the beach and walks barefoot in deep sand until all the numbness and tingling have disappeared. Since I live part of the year near beaches, I frequently walk in the deep sand, gaining all the benefits of fresh air, sea, and sky, beachcombing for shells and driftwood while I treat my feet.

The body, brain, and mind make up an intricate and remarkable interrelating system. With a little attention and with a sense of real appreciation, you can cultivate a new attitude toward your physical self, and feel a new sense of its support in return.

In your notebook:

- Plan the exercise program that is most beneficial for you. Decide what you need most and then devise a realistic program that you can willingly continue week after week.
- Incorporate the following in your exercise program:

  a. Progressive relaxation
  b. Simple stretches
  c. Head rolls and shoulder shrugs
  d. The "chicken wing" for the upper chest
  e. Foot exercises
  f. Your personal choice of pleasurable activity such as easy jogging, fast walking, biking, swimming, low-impact aerobics, or dancing

- Assess the effects of your program. Are you really doing it and how often? Keep a daily record. Do you notice an increased sense of well-being? Are your seizures and their frequency affected?

  Frequency of seizures:

  Severity:

  Type:

  Difference from usual occurrence:

- Do you notice a sense of overstrain? If you do, reduce or alter your program.

- If you find an exercise program difficult to enjoy or maintain, reduce the amount you do or give yourself a day off now and then as a reward or set a goal of doing it only several days a week. Turning exercise for relaxation into stressful achieving simply defeats its purpose.

15

Learning Deep Relaxation

Learning to notice your breathing pattern and being able to change it from tension-producing to relaxation-producing is one of the most crucial—and simplest—mind/body skills.

—Joan Borysenko, Ph.D.[1]

Breathing exercises have been widely practiced for some time now. Shortly after World War II, the European obstetricians Frederick Leboyer and Ferdinand Lamaze became known for teaching deep-breathing techniques to their patients to use during childbirth, making it possible for many women to deliver their babies with little or no anesthesia. The natural childbirth movement grew from this work. At the same time, eastern religious practices were drawing greater and greater attention in the West, but it wasn't until yoga and its forms of meditation became well known that breathing techniques emerged as a central and remarkable force in promoting wellness.

In the United States, popular attention focused on the practice of meditation and breathing for the first time when the Beatles met with guru Maharishi Mahesh. The devotees who followed the Maharishi claimed that their meditational practices brought down their blood pressure. The preventive and curative possibilities for heart disease were immediately apparent. Skeptical at first, medical researchers began to investigate the question of whether or not meditation and the practice of deep diaphragmatic breathing really affected physiological processes. The research was conclusive. Slow, deep breathing not only brought blood pressure and pulse rate down but also created a relaxed and much less anxious state. Today the need for relaxation and the relief of stress are often cited as factors in many diseases and disorders. Stress reduction workshops are now part of many hospitals' outpatient programs, and many corporations offer stress and relaxation training as part of their personnel services.

Most of the early research on stress and deep breathing was in cardiovascular disease, which is not surprising because the heart and its plumbing lend themselves to measurement. This research revealed that stress and its accompanying shallow, upper-chest breathing stimulate the sympathetic nervous system, that chain reaction of nervous and physiological processes that make up the fight-or-flight response. Deep diaphragmatic breathing stimulates the parasympathetic nervous system, another series of nervous and physiological connections that make up what Herbert Benson, M.D., has called the *relaxation response*.

"The Relaxation Response," Dr. Benson writes in *Beyond the Relaxation Response*,[2] "breaks the vicious cycle [of the fight-flight response] by blocking the action of the hormones of the sympathetic nervous system. This blockage prevents anxiety and other harmful effects."

At the Mind/Body Medical Institute, part of Boston's New England Deaconess Hospital and Harvard Medical School, Dr. Benson and his associates conducted a two-year study of relaxation and its effect on seizure occurrence. The number of persons completing the program was not great, but those who stayed with it reduced the number and severity of their seizures.

It is my conviction and also that of Donna Andrews, the epilepsy counselor who works with Joel Reiter, that the practice of deep relaxed breathing is the single most important self-care practice for epilepsy.

Deep relaxed diaphragmatic breathing has immediate beneficial effects. The body warms and relaxes. Panic and shakiness subside. You feel much less anxious. The deep relaxing breaths bring out the life-giving, health-enhancing resources that the body has within itself. You are stimulating its remembered wellness.

Shallow, rapid, upper-chest breathing is recognized as a

cause of seizure activity in the brain. In fact, when you are undergoing an electroencephalogram, the EEG technician will ask you to breathe rapidly. He wants to find out if this breathing brings out a burst of epileptic brain wave activity. It has done so in my case, and it reminds me of my need to keep stress at a minimum and to release it frequently by practicing deep diaphragmatic breathing.

In everyday life, rapid, shallow breathing is usually caused by stressful situations. Some tense persons—and I am one—almost hold their breath in moments of stress. Afterward I feel extra fatigue and shakiness. Others become so habituated to shallow breathing that they are not conscious that they breathe in this way and they are unaware of its costs.

A few individuals in my seizure workshops have been afraid to try deep diaphragmatic breathing, thinking that it will trigger a seizure. It is not likely to happen. Joan Borysenko, formerly head of the Mind/Body Workshops at Harvard Medical School, does not know of any increase in seizures among the people she has encouraged to do deep breathing. Joel Reiter states that hyperventilation brings on petit mal attacks. The slow, deep, diaphragmatic breathing should not.

Deep relaxation does more than create a generalized effect in the body. It can regenerate sexual activity, among other benefits. It is a joke among meditators that they often come out of their period of meditation feeling some sexual arousal. Sex therapists use relaxation techniques in their practice. Some persons with epilepsy experience a sex drive considered much less than normal, and deep relaxation will help to energize it. If you and your partner are happy as is, however, it doesn't matter how "normal" is defined. If you would like to give deep relaxation a try as an aid to sexual activity, tell yourself just before you practice deep diaphragmatic breathing for twenty minutes, "I want to make wonderful love right afterward." Then relax and focus on your breathing. You are likely to find that your body will take care of the rest.

Deep diaphragmatic breathing is a simple and easy

method to learn. You need only yourself to do it. If your support person learns it, too, all the better.

What is deep breathing? It is filling the lungs on the in-breath so full of air that the diaphragm, a balloon-like membrane at the base of the lungs, stretches downward, forcing the abdomen to expand. On the out-breath this muscle goes back into place and then expands into the lung area, forcing air out of the lungs. The belly will then fall slightly.

STEP-BY-STEP INSTRUCTIONS
FOR DEEP BREATHING

1. Lie flat on the floor to make it easier to learn the method. Close your eyes and give your attention to the breath. If you think a seizure might occur, keep your eyes open.

2. Let your hands rest lightly on your abdomen. Exhale, emptying all the air from your lungs. Feel the belly sink slightly. Now breathe in, inhaling until you feel your full lungs pressing against the diaphragm and forcing it to expand into the abdominal cavity, the belly rising. Now exhale, feeling the belly return to normal and your lungs and chest collapse slightly.

3. Now take long, slow breaths. Deep breathing needs to be done slowly for maximum effect. Begin with a count of four or five for each inhalation and exhalation. Count slowly but not uncomfortably so, just slowly enough to make sure that your lungs fill fully and deeply and clear thoroughly.

4. Practice daily or twice daily until deep breathing comes readily and naturally. Set aside ten or fifteen minutes twice a day for a while. Sit down in a comfortable chair, reclining slightly, or lie on the floor or a firm surface. Place a hand on your abdomen to make sure it rises and falls. Concentrate on the breath. Imagine the breath passing into the nose, to the back of the throat, down the passage into the bronchial area, and into the amazing spongy sacks of lungs. Find your own visualization of this process. Keep your attention focused on the breath. When your attention wanders, bring it back gently and visualize the process again.

5. Any exhalation can be used to release tension. When you feel you are tense and under stress, give the out-breath a whoosh to let go of everything. President Jimmy Carter used to do this when he was under fire in a White House press conference. As every basketball fan has observed, a great professional player will stand at the free-throw line and let out a long breath before he makes his throw, almost always sinking the shot. Television close-ups show major-league baseball pitchers letting out a breath just before the pitch, and the Olympic diver Greg Louganis doing the same as he balances on the tip of the board.

I often combine deep diaphragmatic breathing with a walk. Once the rhythm of my pace is established, I coordinate deep inhalations and exhalations with that rhythm, concentrating my attention on maintaining the rhythmic walking and breathing. When my attention wanders and I lose the rhythm, I simply bring myself back and begin again. The benefits are double in half the time. It is always illuminating to notice where my thoughts go when they wander. I make note of the negative, self-critical ones and return to a less anxious, more relaxed, attitude.

It is curious to me that there has not been greater medical and psychological attention given to proper breathing. In purely physiological terms inhalation and exhalation are essential to life and perform the functions of oxygenating the bloodstream and cleansing it of carbon dioxide. Although the airway, bronchii, and lungs are acknowledged and studied in modern medicine, using them in the voluntary/involuntary act of breathing has been neglected. Why this should be so is curious. The word itself suggests its importance. In its Latinate form, *respiration*, it is closely related to spirit and the Latin *spiritus*, the breath of life. We expire with our last breath; we perspire, a kind of breathing through the skin; and we inspire by giving ourselves and others a lift. Through the Latin root, *spirare*, breath, spirit, and hope are intertwined.

In your notebook:

- Practicing deep diaphragmatic breathing:
  Number of minutes each day:
  Monday Tuesday Wednesday Thursday Friday Saturday Sunday

  Be sure to practice daily or twice daily until deepening your breathing pattern is an automatic response to stressful situations.
- How does deep breathing make you feel? Describe as completely as you can.
- Test its effectiveness for you by taking your pulse before and after you practice. This test registers for some persons but not for all. I am able to bring down my pulse rate by ten points with twenty minutes of deep diaphragmatic breathing (not when I'm walking, too, of course). Record your pulse rate and notice the changes. A simple way to take your pulse is to place two fingers on the carotid artery just to the side of the wind pipe in your neck. Count the throbs for sixty seconds.

16

Nutritional Concerns

*My guiding principle is moderation. Except for an absolute
ban on smoking, I am not a fanatic about anything. . . .
Through the principles of moderation . . . [you can] . . .
live healthfully and enjoyably.*

—Jane Brody[1]

Although medical doctors may be skeptical, many
people with epilepsy believe that their seizure occurrences
have a great deal to do with their diet. Not only alcoholic
beverages and other abusive substances affect seizures but
what we eat and don't eat seems to as well. Hippocrates and
his followers used diet therapy in the fourth and third
centuries B.C. to treat epilepsy, but little is done today. There
are two diets recommended in certain cases of epilepsy by
medical doctors. Other than those we are on our own. The
need for solid research here is urgent.

In my view and from my experience, the high-fiber, low-
fat, low-sugar, moderate-protein diet widely accepted at
present should be helpful for people with seizures. High
fiber acts as a control on fluctuations of blood sugar. Preventing glucose highs and lows is important if not critical
for people with epilepsy. In addition, recent and ongoing
research in the brain sciences reveals the roles of certain
brain chemicals and hormones that are metabolized in the
body from certain nutrients, particularly protein. Changes
in the neurophysiological conditions in the body are also
moderated by a nourishing, balanced, regular diet.

SUGAR AND FIBER

Recent research on sugar, fiber, and general diet has changed our views about the connection between what we eat and how our bodies function. Since fluctuations in blood sugar (glucose) may be implicated in seizure conditions, it is important to look at the role of sugar in the diet. Both high blood sugar as in diabetes and low blood sugar as in hypoglycemia are conditions in which seizures or convulsions occur. Although sugar intake is not as critical in epilepsy as in the other two conditions, the general principles for keeping blood sugar levels steady and moderate apply to us.

The principal rules to follow in planning and preparing meals are twofold: fewer processed foods are better and balanced meals keep glucose levels more even, without highs and lows, and within the range of normal. Current research has established sound reasons for recommending less processed foods. In processed foods, those that are canned, powdered, dried, or precooked, the fiber has already been broken down. The digestive system has little to do, and the sugar content is absorbed into the bloodstream rapidly, boosting your glucose level. Foods where the fiber is more intact are absorbed much more slowly. Consequently, the recommended diet today emphasizes fresh foods rather than processed foods; steaming, baking, and stir-frying for vegetables rather than boiling or long cooking methods; baked or steamed potatoes instead of instant ones; unprocessed whole grains and cereals instead of precooked ones; and whole fruits rather than juices.

The important point here is the fiber content. Balanced meals should include both fats (not much) and fiber to slow the digestive process. Fruits and vegetables contain fructose, a simple sugar that can be as readily absorbed as refined sugar. The digestive system must work longer and more slowly on high-fiber foods so that blood sugar (glucose) is released more slowly over a long period, making for a more even rise and fall of glucose levels. The entire digestive tract will be far healthier, and cholesterol levels will be lower with this dietary approach.

High fiber means 20 to 30 grams a day. The book *Your Defense Against Cancer*[2] recommends 30 to 40 grams. And that's a lot of fiber. Most fruits and vegetables have very little—1 to 3 grams. Many commercial breakfast cereals, even the best, yield 2 or 3 grams a serving. The most delicious bran muffin has 2 grams. Short of eating ten or fifteen muffins a day with calories in excess of 3,000, where can we find 20 to 30 grams of fiber? It takes some doing. I manage a 15-gram breakfast with a serving of Kellogg's All-Bran (10 grams) and a banana (3 grams) with a sprinkling of granola for flavor (2 grams). Once I've hit 15 grams, I let the additional grams take care of themselves from whole and lightly cooked foods at the other two meals.

Preventing the glucose highs and lows is the reason behind the recommendation of low consumption of sugar for persons with seizures. The definition of sugar includes honey, maple syrup, and so-called "sugarless" jams and fruit syrups that are sweetened with fructose (fruit sugar).

If you should eat a sweet, be sure that it is with a meal when you are digesting proteins, fats, and fibers. As a between-meal snack a sweet will enter the bloodstream as glucose much more rapidly than it does when it accompanies other foods. When you consume a sweet snack, you can burn it off by exercising immediately afterward.

Canned or processed foods are unavoidable from time to time. You need to become a label reader to avoid those brands that list sugar, corn syrup, corn sweetener, honey, and caramel among their ingredients. Canned fruits marked "lite" contain little or no added refined sugar. They and some fruit juices and jams are sweetened with other fruits that are as rapidly absorbed into the system as cane or beet sugar. However, they are much less sweet to the taste. Once you cut down on your sugar intake, you will notice how excessively sweet many processed and packaged foods are.

Even commercial bread may taste disagreeably sweet to you. Your taste buds will help you eliminate these products from your diet.

I find it hardest to avoid sugar when I need a mid-morning or late-afternoon pickup, and I've learned to keep a packet of dry-roasted nuts in my bag and in my cupboards. They are filling and nutritious, a good source of protein, fat, and fiber, and they keep me away from candy bars, cookies, and those ubiquitous and seductive homemade ice cream parlors.

SPECIAL DIETS

Two special diets have brought considerable relief for some cases of seizures. One of them is the ketogenic diet, and the other is the hypoglycemic diet.

The ketogenic diet is high in fats and low in carbohydrates and produces ketones, or a state of ketosis, in the body. It was prescribed fairly frequently before anticonvulsant medication dominated the scene. The diet's greatest disadvantage is that it requires precise measurement in grams of everything taken into the body. For most of us it is highly impractical. For the mother of a seriously afflicted child whose medication has little effect, this diet is worth the effort. Recent studies show great improvement when it has been strictly followed. Since ketosis needs to be monitored by blood work and urinalysis, this diet requires the supervision of a physician or a nutritionist. Today the use of MCT oil (medium-chain triglycerides in oil form) helps to induce ketosis and makes the food on the diet list more palatable.

Most of us were put through glucose tolerance tests during workups to find causes for our seizures. The reason these tests are done is that low blood sugar or hypoglycemia can cause seizures. These are eliminated when the low blood sugar is corrected by a special hypoglycemic diet. In this diet, starches such as potatoes, pasta, and refined sugar are eliminated, and foods such as meat, fish, nuts, fresh fruits, and vegetables are emphasized. Five or more small meals a day are substituted for the usual three. Your physician or neurologist will recognize hypoglycemia and will prescribe the dietary regimen to correct it.

During my original workup, I passed the glucose tolerance test and was judged not to be hypoglycemic. No special diet has ever been prescribed. I follow a modified version of the recent recommendations for sugar control in diabetes. It is simply good nutrition to keep highly caloric, nonnutritious substances such as sugar and other sweeteners at a minimum and to eat unprocessed fresh or lightly processed fruits and vegetables with the fiber content largely intact. These considerations make for a moderate, easy-to-follow dietary regime that is nutritious and good for the health and normal functioning of the digestive tract. The only adverse effect I have noticed is an occasional yearning for dessert or a sweet. When this happens, once a week or so I give myself a treat, thus avoiding the nagging sense of deprivation that may send the whole regimen down the drain.

NONSUGAR SWEETENERS

Substituting nonsugar sweeteners for refined sugar is not the panacea that it was once believed to be. Saccharin, the original and formerly most popular, was taken off the market for a time because it has been suspected as a possible carcinogen. Today it is back, particularly visible as Sweet'n Low, but it carries a warning on every packet that it is implicated as a cause of cancer.

While saccharin declined in popularity, aspartame became the nonsugar sweetener of choice. Commercially called Nutrasweet and Equal, this substance has been called into serious question by researchers. Some interpreters of the research believe that aspartame may cause brain damage in laboratory animals, whereas others believe that only a very minor portion of the human population, those with a rare genetic disorder, would be affected by aspartame. Recent research at the Massachusetts Institute of Technology suggests that children are vulnerable to adverse effects, but adults probably are not. Those who oppose its widespread use point out that aspartame breaks down in liquids, especially under heat, into ethanol among other substances. Persons who have never had a seizure report seizures after drinking aspartame-sweetened drinks. For those of us with a history of seizures any substance even suspected of adversely affecting brain function is to be avoided.

Other sweeteners such as sorbitol are as high in calories as sugar. Sorbitol, however, is absorbed slowly into the body. It is well to remember that just because the label reads "sugar-free" does not mean that the contents are calorie-free or free of deleterious sweeteners. They are only free of cane or beet sugar.

COFFEE AND TEAS

Coffee and teas play a role in the rise and fall of blood sugar. Caffeine works in the body as a nervous system stimulant that affects the adrenal cortex. Once adrenalin has been released, it activates the liver to secrete glycogen, its stored blood sugar. The rise in blood sugar accounts for the lift coffee and tea give the body. It is the drop later, when the blood sugar is acted upon and brought below normal by the subsequently released insulin, that is dangerous for people with seizures.

Caffeine also constricts the cranial blood vessels. For this reason it is a prominent ingredient in headache remedies, particularly those for migraine. For a person with epilepsy, constricting the blood supply to the brain is absolutely to be avoided.

In spite of caffeine's widespread consumption in our society, there has been little research on its interaction with epilepsy. One research report suggests strongly that caffeine is a proconvulsant, affecting the amygdala deep in the brain, an area implicated in complex partial seizures. In laboratory animals "the neurotoxic effects of caffeine are obvious at high doses" and "a tendency for more severe seizures was noted." The researchers at the University of California–Davis concluded, "Although the doses which prolonged after-discharge duration in this animal model of epilepsy are far greater than those generally consumed by humans, the possibility that caffeine may potentiate human seizures needs further investigation."[3]

This information should be enough to motivate the most inveterate coffee and tea drinker to kick the habit, but it is a hard one to kick. One woman in a seizures workshop weaned herself gradually by mixing caffeinated and decaffeinated coffees as she made her coffee. She gradually increased the decaffeinated. If you can make the break, there are many substitutes on the market today. The variety of fragrant herb teas is almost infinite, and they are carried in most supermarkets. Some herbs contain caffeine, so look on the box for the "no caffeine" label. The new decaffeinated coffees taste almost like the real thing, and most people can't tell the difference between decaffeinated and caffeinated teas. The new cereal grain hot drinks are vastly improved over those available just a few years ago.

Breakfast coffee is the hardest to eliminate or reduce and the most important. Too much morning coffee or coffee on an empty stomach is never a good idea for anyone. Try a grain hot drink with milk. Hot bouillon makes a savory substitute. Campbell's beef and chicken broths are relatively free of sugar and additives, and so are bouillon powders found in health food stores. The commercial cubes contain corn syrup and should be avoided.

Eliminating coffee is very hard for me, but I have cut down substantially to help me go without medication. On days when I feel shaky, I avoid it altogether. On those days, I find it does not taste good. I feel that my body is giving me a warning sign.

Caffeine comes disguised in some medications. Antihistamines, for instance, may contain it to overcome the drowsiness induced by the medication. Sudafed is an over-the-counter antihistamine that is caffeine-free. If you are on an antihistamine or oral decongestant prescription, ask your physician what it contains. If it contains caffeine, ask for a different medication. Caffeine is also an ingredient in diet drinks where it substitutes for sugar. Be sure to read the label before you select a diet drink from the shelves.

An additional reason for avoiding alcohol, caffeine, and sugar is the tendency for some people with seizures to suffer bouts of depression. The fast lift and drop that these substances produce can exacerbate the tendency to depression, which may turn suicidal under certain circumstances. It is wise not to feed this possibility with fast-acting stimulants.

PHYSIOLOGICAL CONDITIONS

Diet can relieve certain physiological conditions that seem to make fertile ground for seizures to occur. Some of these are menstruation and premenstruation, constipation, excessive intake of water, dehydration, and obesity.

MENSTRUATION

Some women experience seizures or an increase in seizure activity during or just before their menstrual periods. The nervous tension and the body's retention of fluids that are part of the premenstrual syndrome seem to affect the occurrence of seizures. All the relaxation exercises and deep diaphragmatic breathing discussed in this book should help to relieve the nervous tension of that time of the month. Whole-grain breads, crackers, and cereals are natural diuretics as is vitamin B_6 and will reduce the body's retention of fluids. Cutting down on all liquids during that period helps, too. See "Special Concerns for Women with Epilepsy" on page 246.

CONSTIPATION

Wilder Penfield, the Canadian neurologist, and others mention constipation as a factor in epileptic conditions. In addition, some anticonvulsants cause constipation. Here again whole-grain foods will help to clear the digestive tract. So will dried fruits—raisins, dates, and apples, in particular. Watch the sugar content here as it is high in dried fruits. Among the fresh fruits, papaya, pineapple, and melon assist in digestion. If you need to resort to a laxative, milk of magnesia is recommended. It is not only a laxative but it brings to the body the trace mineral magnesium believed to help in relieving seizures. Laxatives with psyllium seed husks are effective because they contain 5 grams of fiber per teaspoon.

WATER

The excessive intake of water specified in a currently popular commercial weight-loss program has brought on seizures in three women who previously had them under control by medication. They had been drinking close to a gallon and a half daily. "Excessive water intake is a known trigger for seizures," writes "House Call" columnist G. Timothy Johnson, M.D., in reporting these cases.[4]

Not only will huge amounts of water bring on seizures but so will a condition of extreme dehydration. Both are to be avoided.

When you follow the high-fiber diet, however, you need to drink a reasonable amount of fluids daily. Otherwise, the fiber will absorb too much fluid from your body and rob certain processes like the action of the colon of their needed moisture. Six to eight glasses of water, juices, and herbal teas are recommended.

OBESITY

Obesity, generally speaking, is the least of our problems. Most of us are more often skinny to average in weight, probably because we tend to be tense and "wired." However, some people struggle with excess weight perhaps because of a family pattern. Certain anticonvulsants tend to stimulate weight gain as well. The medication valproate has this effect in some 50 percent of those who take it.

Because obesity contributes to numerous health problems such as heart disease, adult-onset diabetes, and strain on the back, hip, and knee joints, loss of excess weight is better all the way around, but how you lose it is critical for persons with epilepsy.

A gradual loss of weight is the best recommended way of losing it and keeping it off, and it puts the body and nervous system under the least strain. Extreme diets may bring about rapid weight loss, but they also temporarily weaken the body and put it under considerable stress. This additional stress may increase your risk of a seizure. A special caution for epilepsy is to avoid weight-loss diets that call for excessive amounts of water or fluids.

The way of moderation is indicated for people with epilepsy. Staying within the bounds of not-too-much, not-too-little makes for the wisest course in living with a propensity for seizures.

A SUMMARY OF DIETARY GUIDELINES

1. A high-fiber low-fat adequate-protein low-sugar diet is considered the best for optimum health. Current scientific research in nutrition emphasizes the importance of a balance of fiber, protein, and fats. All three are necessary for the body's needs and processes.

2. High fiber means whole grains with the bran left in; fresh vegetables that are lightly cooked by steaming, baking, or stir-frying in vegetable oil or broth; whole fruits rather than juices and fresh fruit rather than canned fruits because the fiber has been broken down in the canning process; brown rice instead of polished white rice. Recommended: 20–30 grams of fiber daily.

3. Low fat means skim milk; reduced use of cooking oils and spreads; removing the skin from chicken before cooking; baking or broiling fish; using lean beef; cutting the fat off lamb; simmering veal in a light tomato sauce, yogurt sauce, or broth. Enough fats will be left for proper metabolism in the body. No more than 30 percent of daily calories, and no less than 15 percent, should come from fats.

4. Moderate amounts of protein mean 3- to 4-ounce servings twice a day. The 16-ounce steaks, half-pound burgers, and half a chicken are things of the past. Animal protein and dairy products supply the eight essential amino acids from which the body metabolizes the additional amino acids that it needs. Since normal brain function depends on certain hormones produced from protein, an adequate supply of protein is important for everyone, but especially for persons with epilepsy. The meat should be lean, skin and fat removed.

5. Low sugar means reducing or eliminating foods that are processed with sugar, corn or maple syrup, corn sweeteners, caramel, honey, and fructose. Whole fruits and vegetables and unsweetened juices contain fruit sugar naturally. Foods sweetened with fructose are preferable to others because they are less sweet to taste and help in changing our need for sweets. Cut down on your use of mixes, processed foods, and canned and dried fruits and vegetables and soups because of their high sugar levels as well as reduced fiber content.

6. If you prefer a vegetarian or almost vegetarian diet, make sure of adequate daily protein through legumes (dried beans, peas, lentils), and/or dairy products. A protein supplement may be needed if you eat little protein from other sources.

7. Eliminate or reduce sources of caffeine.

A WORD ABOUT BREAKFAST

Since breakfast is the most important meal of the day, here are some specific recommendations:

The no-no breakfast: Coffee, sweet roll, and orange juice. This low-fiber, high-sugar (both refined and fructose) plus caffeine combination provides a fast lift and a precipitous drop later, exacerbating the tendency to fatigue, depression, and the possibility of seizure.

The right stuff: Whole (piece of) fruit—half a grapefruit, whole orange, melon, whole-grain cereal with skim milk, no sugar, eggs (only two or three a week as they are high in fats and cholesterol), whole-wheat toast or muffin, corn oil margarine or no-oil spread, decaffeinated coffee or tea, herb tea.

If your seizures occur in the early morning hours, try a whole-grain snack at bedtime: a piece of whole wheat toast or a bran muffin. It may help to keep blood sugar levels more even through the night.

In your notebook:

What you consumed this week:	What you plan to eat:

BREAKFAST

Monday _____

Tuesday _____

Wednesday _____

Thursday _____

Friday _____

Saturday _____

Sunday _____

MID-MORNING SNACK:

Monday _____

Tuesday _____

Wednesday _____

Thursday _____

Friday _____

Saturday _____

Sunday _____

LUNCH:

Monday _____

Tuesday _____

Wednesday _____

Thursday _____

Friday _____

Saturday _____

Sunday _____

MID-AFTERNOON SNACK:

Monday _____

Tuesday _____

Wednesday _____

Thursday _____

Friday _____

Saturday _____

Sunday _____

DINNER:

Monday _____

Tuesday _____

Wednesday _____

Thursday _____

Friday _____

Saturday _____

Sunday _____

- Are you taking in more than a bare minimum of alcohol, caffeine, and/or sugar?
- Are you eating mostly whole grains and less processed foods?
- Do you associate any occurrence of seizures with low points between meals?

Experiment within these guidelines for what is right for you, what makes you feel energized and alert. Some people's digestive systems cannot tolerate unadulterated whole-wheat grains, the chaff on brown rice, or daily servings of legumes. There is no absolutely right diet for all people.

For help with diet and nutrition you may want to consult a specialist. The following agencies can help you in your search: your local chapter of the American Dietetic Association; your local health department; the department of nutrition of a local college, university, or hospital; or the Nutrition Counseling Service, 15048 Beltway, Dallas, Texas, 75234, 1 (800) 527-0227.

17

Supplementary Nutrients

It is the brain which is the messenger to the understanding.

—Hippocrates[1]

Over the past ten years diet has become an accepted part of good health practice. To treat some diseases and illnesses, special diets are prescribed in the course of usual medical treatment. Diets for heart disease, diabetes, and gastrointestinal problems come immediately to mind. Supplementary nutrients, however, are still controversial for most medical practitioners. Whether they do any good or act as placebos is a question not easily answered. In the case of epilepsy, a number of nutrients have been singled out as effective.

The helpful effects of certain nutritional supplements have not been well known either to people with seizures or to most physicians. Only in the last few years as more attention has been focused on nutrition has this information come to light. Today most holistically oriented doctors consider nutrition a principal preventive and curative therapy for many diseases and disorders, one of them being epilepsy.

The supplementary nutrients[2] that have helped relieve seizures for some people are:

Manganese
Vitamin B$_6$
Taurine
Dimethylglycine
Calcium
Vitamin E

Manganese is needed in the body for efficient sugar metabolism, and it is often lacking in modern diets because of its depletion in farmland soils. It is important because it is believed to correct or to help correct the biochemical imbalance present when seizures occur.

Vitamin B_6 is essential for the synthesis of norepinephrine in the brain, and norepinephrine is directly related to feelings of energy and alertness. B_6 is also needed to synthesize taurine.

The amino acid, taurine, occurs naturally in the body as a by-product of metabolism. It is not one of the eight essential amino acids. However, its importance has recently been recognized, and it is now being added to commercial infant formulas such as Similac to make them more equivalent to breast milk, which is rich in taurine. In the brain, taurine helps to stabilize nerve cell membranes and prevent the neurons from sending too many impulses too fast, which is what happens in a seizure. Taurine is closely associated with manganese, and it may work with manganese to alleviate seizure conditions.

DMG (dimethylglycine) occurs naturally in the biochemistry of human metabolism. It is thought to be important in preventing seizures because it enhances oxygen utilization, particularly at the cellular level, with a significant impact on mind and body. Like norephinephrine, it, too, is associated with a feeling of energy and well-being.

Two additional trace minerals are believed by some to relieve seizures. One is zinc, and it is recommended by Carl C. Pfeiffer, M.D., Ph.D., of the Brain Bio Center in Skillman, New Jersey. The other is magnesium. A teaspoon of milk of magnesia three times a day supplies this trace mineral, which is lacking in our diets because of the depletion of it in the soil. Observe your body's response. If diarrhea results (not likely), cut back or discontinue the magnesia.

Calcium's role in seizures is the subject of several current research studies. It figures in the renewal of every cell in the body, and it has a critical role in the brain as part of neurotransmission and in the mechanism of memory. When it is seriously deficient, convulsions may occur. One of the ironies of epilepsy is that anticonvulsant medication inhibits the body's uptake of calcium.

These dietary supplements can be found on the vitamin shelves of many food stores and pharmacies. My personal conviction is that they should be taken under the direction of a nutritionist or physician. Because they are dietary, they must be taken over a long period of time to see if they have an effect on your variety of epilepsy. If they do, they must be continued indefinitely. Such long-term intake, I believe, should be monitored by a trained professional.

When it comes to vitamins, however, most of us throw caution to the winds and pick out what we think we need. If you are of that mind, here are the recommended daily allowances of these supplementary nutrients and their possible side effects:

Manganese: 50–100 milligrams orally at bedtime
Vitamin B_6: 50 milligrams orally each morning
Taurine: 500 milligrams A.M. and P.M.
DMG: 100 milligrams A.M. and P.M.

For some people taurine in such high dosages may give some peptic ulcer distress. It disappears when the taurine is discontinued. Vitamin B_6 has a diuretic effect, and in large doses it can be severely dehydrating, not a good idea for the seizure-prone. There have been numerous reports of individuals taking as much as 500 milligrams daily who have reported difficulty in walking, sensations of electric shock down the spine, and numbness of the feet, hands, hips, lips, and cheek. When they stopped taking vitamin B_6, these symptoms gradually disappeared. If you undertake a regimen of supplementary nutrients, closely monitor your reactions for possible side effects.

Supplementary lecithin requires a special note of caution. Many people take lecithin either under a physician's guidance or from the vitamin counter to eliminate fats and cholesterol from the body. Lecithin is a natural substance that occurs in some plant and animal tissue and in egg yolks. One of its components, choline, is suspect for people with seizures. In laboratory animals, a choline-supplemented diet significantly increased seizures. The researchers concluded, "Our results suggest that supplementation of dietary choline above normal levels might result in increased susceptibility to epileptic seizures. This could result from either a reduced threshold for seizure or from an increase in the rate of seizure development."[3] This conclusion definitely suggests that supplementary lecithin with its choline component is not the treatment of choice for people with seizures.

This research stimulates me to speculate about the future possibility of a dietary method for seizure control instead of the treatment by medication that we have now. Much more research is needed to make this possible; but it is an avenue that should be thoroughly explored.

The following is a checklist of supplementary nutrients:

Vitamin B₆: Lack of B_6 is a recognized cause of seizures particularly among infants and children. Seventy-five milligrams of B_6 daily is administered as therapy. A precautionary adult dosage would be 50–100 milligrams, the amount in most B complex supplements.

Folic acid (part of the B complex): A deficiency may contribute to seizures. It can be repaired by vitamin B complex supplement. A supplement with folic acid is urged for all women who may become pregnant, as it protects against birth defects.

Vitamin B₁₂: Another contributor—when it is lacking, it is also suspected of a role in emotional disorders. B complex supplement restores adequate B_{12} when it is taken daily.

Taurine: Certain essential brain chemicals are metabolized from protein. One of these, taurine, has been taken as a supplemental therapy with success in reducing seizures.

Calcium: Calcium must be present for normal neurotransmissions to take place in the brain. Supplementary calcium (600–1,200 milligrams) helps to guard against dangerously low calcium levels due to anticonvulsant medication.

Vitamin E: Several studies of vitamin E have shown that

400 mg a day give children complete seizure control when it is taken in addition to their medication. Recently, some Finnish research found vitamin E carcinogenic in even small amounts, but this study goes contrary to every other where E has been protective against cancers and enhances the immune system, particularly for the elderly. Further research will no doubt confirm or disprove the Finnish report. Meanwhile, what to do? It's a dilemma. For myself, I have decided to continue with a daily 200 mg of vitamin E.

Trace minerals: Manganese is associated with normalizing neuronal activity in the brain. Magnesium is "able to directly suppress neuronal burst firings and interictal EEG spike generation," says one researcher.

Anticonvulsant medication interferes with the body's absorption of vitamin D, calcium, and folic acid.[4] Supplementary D and vitamin B (folic acid) are needed as well as calcium. A daily multivitamin with a full range of vitamin B including B_6, B_{12}, and folic acid plus minerals is a moderate way to ensure adequate intakes.

If you undertake a program of supplementary nutrients, preferably with a nutritionist or physician, you will need to maintain this experiment for several weeks or months to judge its effectiveness in helping you control your seizures.

Ask yourself and record in your notebook every few days:

1. Do you feel energized and alert?
2. Do you have fewer uppers and downers?
3. Does less fatigue accumulate?
4. Do you get through the day on a more even keel?
5. Are you sleeping more soundly and waking more rested?
6. Are your seizures and preseizure activity less frequent and/or less severe?

Again, these nutrients help some people. Their use, in my view, should be monitored by a nutritionist or a doctor. If your answers are yes, or mostly yes, then your program of supplementary nutrients is helping you. You may notice positive responses to questions 1 through 5 without there being much effect on your seizures. I would suggest staying with your program, anyway. General good health is desirable, and it may affect your seizure frequency over a long period of time.

18

Abusive Substances

When I stopped drinking, when I stopped smoking so much, when I began to think . . . Good Lord, the depression and the prostration of it! . . . All the same, I am better than I was in Paris . . . by eating hardly any solid food and hardly drinking I am pretty weak, but my blood is getting healthier instead of getting poisoned.

—Vincent van Gogh[1]

Vincent van Gogh, the great artist who is believed to have had epilepsy, was a minute and perceptive observer of himself. He recognized not only the terrible bouts of depression that eventually led to his suicide but also the debilitating effects of his life-style: the heavy drinking, smoking, and poor diet that contributed to his difficulties.

Today drinking, smoking, and poor diet along with lack of exercise and obesity make up the five most prevalent destroyers of good health, and they are recognized as such by the medical profession. We have discussed diet, exercise, and obesity in earlier chapters. For people with epilepsy the use of abusive substances—alcohol, cigarettes, and hard drugs—may have serious and possibly fatal consequences.

ALCOHOL

Alcohol's effect on epilepsy is now a question. For years it was generally considered to be a stimulant to seizure activity, and persons with epilepsy were urged by their physicians and neurologists to abstain completely. More recent studies, particularly those done by Richard Mattson, M.D., of Yale University School of Medicine, indicate a more flexible approach. A summary of his studies appeared in a recent Epilepsy Foundation of America newsletter.

> Those studied who had one drink on a single social occasion (which he characterized as "very light drinkers") had no increased risk of seizures; those who had one to two drinks ("light drinkers") had a 5 percent risk of increase in seizures; those who drank two to three drinks ("moderate drinkers") had a 17 percent increased risk of seizures; those who drank five or six drinks ("moderate-heavy drinkers") had a 58 percent increased risk of seizures and people with epilepsy who drank more than six drinks ("heavy drinkers") had an 80 percent increased risk of seizures.[2]

In addition, Dr. Mattson finds that additional abuses put certain persons at greater risk of seizures when they are drinking.

> People who drink to excess often have poor eating habits, don't get enough sleep, and have a number of other illnesses tied to alcohol abuse, such as hypoglycemia and electrolyte imbalance, which may result in seizures.
>
> People who drink to excess are predisposed to head trauma and infection, which in turn may cause seizures.
>
> Some people have both epilepsy and alcoholism. In some cases, the epilepsy predates the alcoholism and in some cases it follows it. People who develop epilepsy after years of drinking are then susceptible to seizures even during periods of abstention from alcohol.
>
> Sporadic, moderate to heavy drinking, particularly when combined with loss of sleep, may be followed by isolated seizures the next morning and may be a sign of latent epilepsy.
>
> Seizures may be precipitated in nonalcoholic people with epilepsy by moderate use of alcohol, especially during the six to twenty-four hours after drinking.[3]

An additional caution, according to the *Physicians Desk Reference* for prescription drugs, is that the anticonvulsant Dilantin (phenytoin) should not be combined with alcohol.

In my own case I find that even one glass of wine with dinner every night puts me at high risk, particularly if other circumstances are stressful as well.

How does an alcoholic drink affect the system? Recently the *Tufts University Diet and Nutrition Letter* carried a short description headlined "From the mouth to the brain." It said:

> Unlike protein, fat, and carbohydrate, all of which must pass from the stomach to the small intestine before being absorbed into the bloodstream, about 20 percent of the alcohol we drink goes directly from the stomach to the blood. . . . Most of the remaining alcohol goes through the small intestine. Once in the bloodstream, the body handles alcohol [ethanol] much as it would a drug, quickly setting about its elimination. About 3 percent leaves the body unmetabolized via urine, perspiration, and expired air. The rest, formerly thought to be almost exclusively metabolized by the liver, is now believed to be processed in significant amounts in the stomach and small intestine right after it is consumed. Since the intestine can only work on about 7 grams of alcohol (about a quarter of an ounce) an hour, it starts to accumulate in the bloodstream and affect other organs, notably the brain. . . . In the brain, alcohol acts as a narcotic, actually putting nerve cells "to sleep." This anesthetic effect begins in areas of the brain that control behavior. . . . As blood alcohol levels rise, other brain centers become depressed.[4]

This pathway is the one by which alcoholic beverages affect normal people with more or less normal brain function. In one research study the normal participants were given EEGs after drinking alcoholic beverages, and half of them showed epileptic brain wave patterns. Alcohol's effect on the neurons of people prone to seizures is likely to be even more dramatic. Control of erratic swift firing of neurons is made exceedingly difficult. Accidents, both minor and automotive, are more likely to happen. Alcohol dehydrates the body and inhibits the absorption of vitamins A, B, and

C. With extremely heavy use brain cells are irreversibly damaged.

It is easier to get along without alcohol than you may think at first. There is no doubt that social drinking is almost universal, but not drinking is no longer as odd as it used to be. One possible substitute is a drink made with mineral water or quinine water on ice with a lemon twist. It looks like vodka or gin, and you will find that you don't really miss the taste or the calories from the alcohol. Today there are also many nonalcoholic substitutes available at natural food stores and many supermarkets. As a substitute for wine you can choose from a wonderful array of fruit juices, some of them made from wine grapes. Nonalcoholic wine and beer are also readily available. To produce nonalcoholic wine the wine is made by the usual process, and then the alcohol is removed. A trace, perhaps as much as 1 percent, may remain. Club soda with some flavor or fruit juice added, a "spritzer," is always good. Nonalcoholic champagne and sparkling apple ciders are on the market, too. Soft drinks are not a good substitute because of the sugar and caffeine content in many of them.

SMOKING

Smoking does not have the direct and dramatic effect on the brain that alcohol has. However, it undermines good health practices. Particles in smoke combine with other molecules to reduce the blood's supply of oxygen, an absolute necessity for every body and brain function. The brain's neurons require a steady and consistent supply of oxygen to function normally. Smoking dehydrates the body as alcohol does. It is a primary cause of lung cancer, second after heart disease as a cause of death.

This addiction is extremely hard to break and gets harder as the years go by. It is beyond the scope of this book to give in detail methods to break the smoking habit, but the excellent book, *Your Defense Against Cancer*, by Henry Dreher,[5] lays out effective strategies step-by-step.

DRUGS

Recent research indicates that marijuana has an injurious effect on the brain. When the active ingredient in marijuana was injected into laboratory rats over half their lifespan, they suffered a loss of some 20 percent of their brain cells. Comparable loss in humans, researchers believe, would affect memory and emotions adversely, producing the effect of premature aging.[6] In Dr. Joel Reiter's clinical experience, however, he finds that "small amounts of marijuana are probably less harmful than small amounts of alcohol for people with seizures."

Harder drugs are another matter."I consider cocaine and amphetamines dangerous in even small amounts for people with seizures," Joel Reiter states. Current studies confirm his view. "Cocaine," it is reported, "has the potential to produce seizures and panic reactions,"[7] even when it is taken in small amounts or only once. Death may be the result. It is painfully obvious these are substances to be avoided by everyone but especially by people with epilepsy.

The primary lesson in self-care is to listen to what your own body tries to tell you. When you feel funny or shaky, when you experience your aura, or when you are in circumstances that have induced a seizure in the past, then be sure to avoid all the substances discussed here.

In your notebook:

- Observe and make notes on your own responses to alcohol and its effect on the frequency and severity of your seizures. Notice particularly if alcoholic beverages alone affect you or if their injurious effects occur along with other circumstances and conditions such as stress and tension, ill health, or menstruation. Plan a program to alleviate these conditions and give it in detail here.
- What is your experience with smoking? If you smoke, have you tried to quit and lost the battle? Consult the book, *Your Defense Against Cancer,* for help in designing a program for quitting.
- If you are a user of marijuana, what is your experience with its effect on

your seizures? If they increase in number or severity, make notes here on ways to reduce or eliminate its use.

- If you use cocaine or amphetamines, seek help to break these habits, as they are potentially fatal. Consult your physician, neurologist, or local drug abuse agency. Write down their names, addresses, and telephone numbers here. Make note of their comments and your feelings and responses to them. Being aware of your own willingness or resistance will help you to make good use of their help.

19

Environmental Hazards

Exposure to toxic materials is an ever-growing hazard of civilized existence. . . . Permanent or temporary nervous system damage is one of the most severe consequences.

—Christopher G. Goetz et al.[1]

A doctor is made strangely ill by the pesticide sprayed in her summer cottage to eradicate carpenter ants. Laws require buildings to remove the asbestos once used as insulation and fireproofing. Some 3,450 children of 69,000 tested over a two-year period have "blood-lead concentrations in the potentially toxic level." A neurologist testifies that the accused's violent behavior can be caused by toxic chemicals.

If we read or listen to the news these days, we are treated to such items as the above, and these are only a selection. The pervasiveness of exposure to toxic chemicals makes it difficult not to feel helpless about protecting ourselves and our children. The underfunded and restricted federal and state agencies charged with environmental protection are enough to make the most optimistic person a depressed cynic. Nonetheless, being informed helps. There is good news, too. The damage done to the nervous system can in many cases be reversed.

What should persons with epilepsy look for? There are two major categories: heavy metals and pesticides.

HEAVY METALS

Most of us are aware of the hazards of lead poisoning. One of the success stories in cleaning up the environment is the removal of lead from gasoline, thereby cutting significantly the amount of organic lead that we inhale and absorb. Paint and putty made of lead are no longer widely sold. The danger arises from the residues of old paint and glazing compound in old houses, school buildings, and apartments. The old lead-based paint powders and flakes, or it is dispersed through the air when window sills and other surfaces are sanded. Pieces of old glazing compound loosen and fall to the floor where toddlers can find them and put them into their mouths. Pregnant and nursing mothers can transmit lead to the fetus or infant. A lead compound was once used to relieve sore nipples for nursing mothers!

The lead[2] is carried throughout the body in the bloodstream. Even though the blood tends to eliminate its burden of lead, the amount lodged in the brain remains relatively stable, and in high concentrations exhibits its damaging effects on the nervous system. The symptoms among children resemble epilepsy with headache, trembling of facial muscles, ringing in the ears, and generalized convulsions. Adults notice something going wrong with their hands and feet as well as experiencing unsteadiness in movement. Seizures may occur. For anyone who already has seizures the increased risk is apparent.

If you suspect lead poisoning, you should consult your physician immediately. Many children's hospitals have poison emergency centers. There is effective treatment available. Lead can be removed from brain and body through the process of chelation. In chelation certain chemicals are injected into the body. These bind with the lead and are excreted mainly through the urine. This process is not entirely benign and painless, but it is the treatment of choice.

A certain amount of prevention may be possible through diet. A high-fat, low-mineral, low-protein or high-protein diet increased lead absorption in one research study[3] whereas a high-mineral diet decreased it. Supplementary iron seems to make a difference in lowering retention of lead in the body. Beta-carotene, the food precursor of carotene, and vitamin C are notable dietary chelating elements and are highly recommended as actors on various pollutants roaming the body. These are preventive measures and should not be considered with serious lead poisoning.

Other heavy metals also affect the nervous system. Mercury[4] is absorbed into the brain, damaging the blood-brain barrier in the process. Aluminum[5] accumulates in certain parts of the brain and is noted in the autopsies of Alzheimer's disease patients. How do we avoid these damaging or potentially damaging substances? Unless we are workers in certain industries where we are exposed to them, our absorption of many will be minimal. In the case of aluminum, it is widely used in common household and personal care items and is much harder to avoid. It is not directly implicated in seizures, but its potential damage to the brain or nervous system suggests that it should be avoided, if possible. Here are some suggestions for eliminating aluminum from every day use:

1. Eliminate commonly used products that contain aluminum. Some of these are Bufferin and other brands of painkillers that are buffered with aluminum, deodorants that contain aluminum as a drying agent (all the "super-dry" and "extra-dry" versions), and antacids such as Rolaids. (Tums does not contain aluminum.)

2. Eliminate commonly used foodstuffs that contain aluminum. Table salt is one. All the well-known brands contain aluminum to keep the salt dry. One brand that is aluminum-free is Westbrae (found in health food stores). Sea salt is another. Some baking powders and some self-rising flours also contain aluminum.

3. Become a label reader. Ingredients must be listed on the labels of all foodstuffs. If aluminum is on the list, search out a substitute.

For a while aluminum pots and pans and bakeware were suspect as sources of aluminum taken into the body. Recent research, according to the *Tufts University Diet and Nutrition Letter*, exonerates aluminum cookware from this charge. The new pans, however, come with a protective, nonstick coating.

PESTICIDES AND OTHER CHEMICALS

The term *pesticides* includes insecticides, fungicides, and herbicides. These toxic substances are so widely and persistently used by modern agriculture and industry that it will take the most vigorous public campaign to limit and reduce their use. Most of us use household and garden products that are small-package versions of many of these toxic chemicals. Even when we do so only from necessity when all else has failed, we then have the containers to dispose of in some manner that doesn't contaminate the air, soil, and water. These environmental pollutants pose one of the most difficult dilemmas of the present day and many days to come.

For people with epilepsy, already trying to manage a sensitized nervous system, the problem is acute. We are particularly vulnerable to these substances. One woman with seizures wrote to me:

> I was sure some reaction to pesticides was wrong with me. I was in a doctor's office and . . . bit into an orange I'd picked up in a recently sprayed orchard, ate some of the peel and went into what became a classic pattern of unpleasant events.

In a recent murder case the neurologist David Bear[6] appeared as an expert witness for the defendant, a man without a previous record of violence who had been working for a chemicals company. Dr. Bear testified that the carbaryl (over-the-counter insecticide Sevin) that the accused had been mixing and applying, could affect the brain's regulatory mechanisms, the amygdala and the hippocampus, so that an uncontrollable violent act was indeed possible.

"Preexisting neurologic disease," state three researchers, "may be exacerbated or accentuated following exposure to some offending materials."[7] The warning for adults and children with seizures is clear.

Pesticides and other chemicals affect the nervous system by two routes. One is massive exposure or ingestion, when an acute toxic reaction occurs. Treatment should be immediate in a hospital where laboratory testing can pinpoint the offending chemical and the victim can be monitored by physicians and medical technicians.

The second route, more insidious and difficult to detect, is low-level exposure over an extended time period. This process is called *kindling* and is the basis for the current laboratory research on chemicals and seizures. "Many of the characteristics of human epilepsy," Mary E. Gilbert, Ph.D. writes, "are present within the kindling model, including, for example, its initially focal origin, reduction in threshold with ensuing convulsive attacks, permanency, its response to anticonvulsant therapy, and the presence of interictal . . . signs of enhanced excitability."[8]

In the animal experiments conducted by Mary Gilbert and others, the development of seizures consistently followed repeated low-level injections of several classes of pesticides. Once this degree of sensitization to seizures has been reached, further seizures occurred more readily. The chlorinated hydrocarbon insecticides lindane and dieldrin are "the most effective and consistent potentiators [of kindling acquisition]," according to Robert M. Joy,[9] another researcher. Mary Gilbert has found that the formamidine insecticides amitraz and chlordimeform increase kindled seizures that originate in the amygdala and hippocampus deep in the limbic area of the brain. Dr. Gilbert's current research concentrates on another class of pesticides, the pyrethroids, that interfere with biochemical interactions in the brain and produce seizures,[10] although she believes them to be less neurotoxic than the others. Synthetic pyrethroids, the most potent, are used in flea powders and shampoos. Pyrethroids account for 30 percent of the world's pesticides.

Because kindling "appears to be a universal property of nervous systems,"[11] the research done with laboratory animals can be extrapolated to humans. Mary Gilbert points out that developing organisms are the most at risk to neurotoxic effects. Children are especially vulnerable. She says, "Chronic low-level exposure may be more detrimental than exposures that produce overt seizures from onset."[12]

What can we do to protect ourselves and children from

neurotoxic pesticides and chemicals? Avoiding them entirely is the best course. If you must use them, wear protective clothing and wash your hands and face and any exposed skin afterwards. Do not use them inside the house. For house plants, simply pick off the insects. When ants or other insects invade, have someone else do what spraying may be indicated outside the house, not inside where the spray residue will be contained. These are prudent precautions for everyone. Pesticides that were once considered safe for over-the-counter sale are being reassessed, and a number of them are being withdrawn from the market. They are not to be used without serious thought. Reading the labels before use is mandatory. As you read, look for the chlorinated hydrocarbons, lindane and dieldrin, and the formamidines, chlordimeform and amitraz, as the basic chemicals. These offenders have been thoroughly researched for their serious neurotoxicity.

In your notebook:

- Go through your household and garden chemicals to discover what you are using. Read the labels for their chemical composition.
- For what purposes are you using these chemicals? Find substitutes or think of ways to do without them.
- Have you ever noticed a relationship between pesticide use and your seizures or changes in behavior that are uncharacteristic of you? Describe what happened and what chemical you used or had used by others. Discuss this incident with your neurologist.

PART SIX

USING
INTERVENTIONS

20

Stopping Seizures by Yourself

It has been repeatedly observed, since ancient times, that a specific sensory stimulus could arrest epileptic fits. . . . This phenomenon of seizure-arrest, known for so long, has not been seriously investigated in the laboratory or clinic. . . . This neglect is surprising since a study of naturally arrested seizures is both of theoretical interest and pertinent to therapy.

—Robert Efron, M.D.[1]

As I settled into the circle at the first meeting of a support group for persons with seizures, I realized that the man to my left suffered from what these days are called developmental disabilities. Usually we don't see retarded people at meetings, and I was immediately impressed by the simple courage it took for him to be there, accompanied by his mother and the director of the group home where he lived. As the discussion turned to methods we can use to help ourselves, particularly dispelling fear, he spoke and I was impressed even further. "I do that," he said, his voice somewhat hoarse and halting. "I tell myself, keep calm, keep calm."

"Does the seizure stop?" I asked.

He nodded. "It goes away," he said.

"Did someone teach you to do that?" I asked.

He shook his head, looking a little hurt. "I thought of it myself," he said.

I turned away in wonder, impressed that even a person whose functioning was as compromised as his had found a way to intervene on his own behalf and arrest a seizure. This man's personal experience was an addition to the growing number of similar accounts that I had heard since reading Dr. Efron's case history of the woman who aborted her seizures with a sniff of jasmine. The literature of epilepsy as Dr. Efron notes in the quotation at the beginning of this chapter is scattered with examples of "naturally arrested seizures." The neurosurgeon Wilder Penfield records a number of instances in his book, *Epilepsy and the Functional Anatomy of the Human Brain*.[2]

My own experience and that of others in the Mind/Body Workshops now at the New England Deaconess Hospital in Boston confirms these cases. When I began to present workshops for people with seizures in the Boston area, I taught the methods for the natural arrest of seizures that I had learned from this literature and from experience. Some participants had already discovered their own methods, but they had never used them systematically. Others learned new methods and, using them at the right moment, found them effective in stopping a seizure.

Using any method to arrest a seizure depends on your recognizing your typical aura, the preliminary event that signals the onset of a seizure. Return to chapter 11 and review the kinds of auras and the ways to recognize them. Reread your notes on that chapter to remind you of your own personal experiences of an aura. Once you recognize your aura, you can act in time to abort a seizure.

USING SENSORY STIMULI

Sensory stimuli make up the largest category of methods of natural arrest, probably because many auras are experienced as distinct sensations. Dr. Efron commented in his article, "The Conditioned Inhibition of Uncinate Fits," that both processes, that of precipitating a seizure and that of arresting a seizure, "must represent converse aspects of the process of excitability of neural tissue."[3] If a seizure is preceded by a smell, for example, then another smell may arrest it.

Commenting on "Sensory Arrest," Wilder Penfield wrote, "When an attack is just beginning, strong stimulation of the part threatened may avert the further development of a seizure."[4]

When the uncus, a kind of beak on the hippocampus in the limbic area of the brain where odors are processed, is involved, the aura will be a smell, and a smell will be used in the arresting procedure. In his study of the woman who sniffed jasmine, Dr. Efron reported that his patient had discovered that she could arrest a developing seizure by inhaling the unpleasantly strong odor at an early stage in her aura. Although "no arrested seizures had ever occurred" in twenty-six years of epilepsy, once she began to use the powerful scent, Dr. Efron wrote, "the patient has been able to arrest every seizure by inhaling from the vial the odors of various aromatic chemicals or essential perfume oils."[5]

Recently, Dr. Efron was called in on the case of a young woman whose seizures were not controlled by high levels of medication. The drugs had begun to affect her liver and the ability of her blood to clot, both life-threatening developments. Once again the antidote of inhaling an intense odor succeeded. Her seizures were arrested, and her medication doses could be reduced.

Touch is another sensation effective in stopping a seizure. "In a child of six years," Dr. Efron noted, "his mother found that his focal, adversive attacks which are followed by complete immobility can be arrested by tickling him at the onset of the adversive [turning the head] movement. Sometimes his fits stop when he sees his mother approach to tickle him."[6] This instance is particularly notable because the child learns to stop his seizure sequence on his own!

A taste of something can be employed as an arresting procedure. One of Dr. Efron's patients took a bite of chocolate, and the seizure did not develop. Sugar alone was not effective, Dr. Efron noted. The efficacy of chocolate but not sugar points up the need for you to experiment to find what works for you. If you experience taste or a gastric sensation as an aura, eating something, perhaps a piece of candy, would be a method to try.

Sounds both precipitate seizures and block their development. For example, a musicogenic seizure (one preceded by hearing music, real or imagined) may be arrested by music. A music therapist told me of her client whose brief absence spells were triggered by the calming music the therapist used to help her clients relax. By using a more rousing music she was able to block her client's episodes. Later she met her client outside the office and noticed her slipping into inattention, and she called out to her, "Remember the music! Remember the music!" The woman did and stopped her seizure from going further. Like the child who anticipated being tickled and others who use mental imagery she was able to imagine the music and make it as effective as hearing it in reality.

Tingling sensations are commonly experienced, sometimes in a part of the body, sometimes in the whole body, as part of a seizure. When the tingling begins in a hand or in one arm or leg, you can quickly apply a ligature just above the line where the tingling sensations stop but in the direction where they are headed. This pressure seems to create a barrier, not in the arm or leg but in the region of the brain involved in control of that arm or leg. "The *application of a ligature*," Wilder Penfield comments [italics his], "above the part convulsed, is a method of arrest first said to have been used by Pelops, the master of Galen [the Greek physician of the second century A.D.]."[7] Another variation is to use pin pricks quickly done above the line of tingles. There is no need to draw blood. The sensory stimulus will have the same effect as the ligature.

Early one morning, my most vulnerable time, I felt powerful tingling sensations pervading my entire body. Were they indicative of a seizure's onset? I was immediately frightened and told my husband who was in the room what I was feeling. "Get up and move around," he suggested. At first I resisted. Whether this resistance was the stage in a seizure when movement is impossible or was a psychological resistance, I am not sure, but as soon as I was aware of resisting, I stood up and moved around. The tingling subsided, and no seizure developed.

Movement is a common way to arrest a seizure, perhaps because it is easily done on your own. One of Dr. Efron's early patients moved quickly to put his head between his legs, and another got up and walked around, blocking his seizure from developing. Another neurologist who has done research in self-arrest of seizures noted that several people in his study increased physical activity as a method. One man said he hollered, beat on himself, and moved around while another "moves around and slaps [his] arms."[8] "In a . . . motor seizure," Dr. Penfield writes, "the subject often seizes the moving part to hold it still, slaps it, places it in cold water. The patient who suffers from simple adversive seizures [those where the head turns away] without early loss of consciousness may use his hands to turn his head forcibly in the opposite direction."[9] Dr. Efron had a patient whose family members acted quickly in the same manner to abort the seizures they saw beginning.

Sensory stimulation or movement probably are most effective when they are used to arrest seizures that begin with strong sensations or trembling. However, moving around or walking it off seems to be effective in other types of seizures as well.

Almost everyone who has seizures has had the experience of stopping a seizure from developing or of holding it off for a certain period. The important points here are to recognize your experience, to know your typical aura, and then to use your personal method not just once in a while but systematically.

USING THE IMAGING POWERS OF THE BRAIN

No aspect of epilepsy reveals its intimate connection between mind, brain, and body as clearly as the use of mental images to arrest seizures. One particularly dramatic example was presented in the journal *Annals of Neurology*. It read in part:

> He [one research subject] continued to have occasional seizures over the next five years, but he developed a technique

that, when applied at the onset of the aura, appeared to abort the seizure and prevent the convulsive component. As the aura began, he sought privacy, closed his eyes or blinked them rapidly, and imagined himself fishing, his favorite leisure pursuit. The mental imagery was so realistic that he could actually "feel the fish on the pole."[10]

The man discussed in this remarkable article suffered from seizures following surgery for an aneurysm in the brain. Once it had been removed, his seizures began, a common aftermath of brain surgery. His seizures were of the grand mal type, generalized tonic-clonic, and they were preceded by a musical aura. Once the patient knew what the aura signaled, he developed his imaginary fishing trip and was able to arrest subsequent seizures.

What is even more astonishing than the patient's blocking his seizures with mental imagery is that the neurologists observed the mental imagery's effect in eliminating seizure spikes on the man's electroencephalogram. They reported:

> During EEG monitoring, which showed right temporal spikes and sharp waves at 35 to 40 per minute, he simulated the exercise [going fishing] and discharges ceased for as long as three minutes. No change in discharge frequency occurred while he played cards, listened to music, read, or performed mental arithmetic.[11]

The fact that "discharges ceased for as long as three minutes" suggests a remarkable ability inherent in a mental image. There are very few seizures that last more than a minute or two, although the aftermath, sleep or a period of semiconscious recuperation, may extend what looks and feels like part of the seizure. A mental image that blocks the sudden discharges in the brain is a powerful image indeed.

Different from Dr. Efron's female patient who was able to stop her medication, this man, the researchers state, "has continued to take [Dilantin] and to use his imagery technique and has remained . . . free of seizures for three years."[12] When a seizure threatens to break through, it is preceded by the musical aura, and the man knows it is time to take his mental fishing trip.

What is mental imagery that it can have such an effect on the neurochemical processes of the brain? How does it work? Mental imagery is our capacity to imagine and to be conscious that what we imagine does not exist in the world immediately before us. That mental imagery affects the neurochemistry of the brain and body has been widely recognized in the last few years. Once we are conscious of these changes, we can see them occur.

Think about a lemon, for example. Think about its appearance, its feel in your hand, its smell, its taste, its juice in your mouth. Most of us begin to salivate at the mention of the word *lemon*. It is the classic demonstration of the body's response to imagination. We all know what a nightmare does to us. Our hearts pound, our breathing is quick and shallow, we try to move, as if we were threatened in reality by our nightmare images. The thought of making love or the mental image of an absent lover arouses us, stimulating certain biological responses, and putting us in a receptive mood and condition.

When Dr. Efron taught his patient how to imagine the smell of jasmine in time to stop a seizure, he was teaching her through a series of repeated, specific lessons how to imagine the smell of jasmine on a reliable basis. This process is called *conditioning*, and it has been used in many animal experiments. The most famous are those of Ivan Petrovich Pavlov, a Russian physiologist and researcher of the late nineteenth and early twentieth centuries. Human beings are capable of using mental imagery with greater complexity and subtlety than other animals.

The techniques of biofeedback demonstrate the power of mental imagery. These use recording devices to show us how our bodies are affected by what we think and feel. For example, when we are tense and anxious, our hands and feet will be colder then when we are relaxed and at ease. A little thermometer or a temperature sensitive dot of paper will show how we warm our extremities as we relax. In another biofeedback test (galvanic skin response) the skin responds to emotional stimuli from words and names and tasks. The pores open and close almost instantaneously to a spoken word, which is the basis of the lie detector, a device that was developed from the word-association experiments done by Freud and the Swiss psychologist, C. G. Jung, in the early part of this century. Most recently, the electroencephalogram has been used to show a person the alterations of brain wave frequency that occur in different stages of alertness, repose, and sleep. These, too, can be altered at will. The role of this form of biofeedback in controlling seizures is discussed by Dr. Joel Reiter in chapter 22.

The sum of the research in natural arrest of seizures is that our bodies tell us something that most of us do not realize: We have and can exert much more control over our neurophysiological states than was once thought possible.

A mental image may be a picture or a sensation or a thought or a feeling, and all of these have been used by people to stop a seizure in its tracks. In the case of the man who goes fishing, it is a vivid picture with sensory aspects. He can "feel the fish pulling on the pole." For the woman who sniffed jasmine, it is a smell. When the retarded man told the group that he "thinks calm," it is a thought/feeling as it is when deep diaphragmatic breathing induces relaxation. Then we are giving ourselves subtle instructions to be calm and relaxed. When the psychotherapist called out to her client to "remember the music," she remembered the rousing music, a mental image of a sound, something we do every time we try to think of a song or a dance tune, and she blocked her seizure. I can imagine the priest/healer at the Asklepion of Epidaurus saying to N. N. from Argos, "Now, when you feel a seizure coming on, remember the ring that the god Asklepios pressed against your mouth, nostrils, and ears in your dream." The power of that image would surely block a seizure if going fishing will do it.

My first experience of arresting a seizure with a mental image occurred during the course of the Mind/Body Workshop in the Department of Behavioral Medicine at Harvard Medical School. Instructed by Joan Borysenko, Ph.D., and Steve Maurer, I had learned the effective stress-relieving method of deep diaphragmatic breathing and was practicing it daily in twenty-minute meditations. Midway through the workshop I found myself having a series of brief seizures, ones without unconsciousness and convulsion. Each episode, a sudden surge of sensation up the back of my head, was accompanied by intense fear. I panicked at first and did not think of the deep breathing. When I did, I sat down and closed my eyes, tried to relax, and began to breathe deeply as the surging sensation began. The seizure itself did not stop, but the feeling of fear was dispelled instantly. I sat still, my eyes closed, my breathing slow and deep, and I watched in my mind's eye as the episode came and went.

Visible in my mind and rising with the surging sensation, a pale gray smoke as if from a fire inside rose up my left leg and through my body, until the smoke hovered over my left shoulder, making a free-form knot. Then it subsided down the same pathway. Not only did I find the experience interesting but afterward I felt no mental confusion or physical exhaustion. That particular kind of seizure has occurred only once in more than five years since, and then it was much milder and fewer episodes occurred. By giving my body the images and signals for relaxation, rather than for fear and anxiety, I seem to have disconnected the neurological sequence for that kind of seizure.

Another participant in the Mind/Body Workshop, a young man of about thirty, had frequent seizures that began with an aura of intense fear and ended in massive convulsions. During the workshop he found that he could arrest a seizure, in the preliminary stages when he was terrified, by using the deep diaphragmatic breathing. He, too, employed the method spontaneously without knowing that it had worked effectively for me. Since then he has used the technique and succeeded in aborting other seizures.

The mental image of relaxation and calmness is immediately formed by the desire to use the deep diaphragmatic breathing. This image then sends its neurochemical consequences through the body.

In the first Boston-area workshop that I led for persons with seizures a woman participant had a similar experience.

Before I presented intervention methods to the group, Martha was alone at an evening meeting and began to feel the strange and "spacey" feelings she recognized as her aura. She panicked with the typical epileptic terrors—how to get home to safety, how to keep it from happening in public. Without a driver's license or a companion she was stranded at the public meeting. Then she remembered the deep breathing that I had taught the group. "I just concentrated on my breathing," she told me later. "I told myself, just relax, be calm. And I took one slow, deep breath after another. The seizure developed to a certain point, then it stopped as if it couldn't go any further—like it was blocked. Then, after a while, it went away. I don't think anyone at the meeting knew what I was going through."

Anger is another thought/feeling that seems to arrest the onset of a seizure. Standing at her kitchen counter one morning Martha felt again the strangeness and spaciness of her aura. "It just made me mad," she told me later. "I just yelled at myself, you can't do this to me, I won't allow it, and the seizure didn't go any further." One teenager reported to a neuropsychologist that he yells "F*** off!" to his seizure and seems to block it.

At the 1988 convention of the American Psychiatric Association, the neurologist Kiffin Penry,[13] whom many consider to be the leading epileptologist in the United States, reported the case of a young woman whose grand mal seizure was recorded on videotape. When she was shown the tape, she responded, "It makes me so ashamed. I'm not going to have any more of those." "And she didn't," Dr. Penry commented. Although this occurrence is not strictly speaking a response to a mental image, the video obviously stimulated a complex inhibitory (and very effective) response.

In 1976, two neurologists, Robert Feldman and N. N. Paul, observed the reduction of seizures in persons who watched their own videotapes and reported:

[Videotapes] provided a means by which patients could acquire otherwise unrecognized or forgotten information. Once equipped with the identity of the specific emotional trigger, the patient could avoid the kind of events which might . . . induce a seizure and . . . [could] cope with environmental cues.[14]

Today videotaping and TV monitoring are routinely employed during a patient's hospital workup for epilepsy. Both Dr. Penry's experience and the earlier use by Doctors Feldman and Paul suggest that using videotape will help a person to recognize his aura or an emotional trigger. Certain kinds of events—the exacerbating circumstances discussed earlier—could be avoided. The powerful effect of seeing yourself in the throes of a seizure may block the seizure sequence in the brain. This method needs to be explored further.

Dr. Pritchard and the others who recorded the effects of the fishing imagery concluded that seizures originating from a focus in the right hemisphere of the brain are most amenable to being blocked by an image. The right hemisphere has a greater role in visual imagination than the left. Four persons in that study had right-hemisphere foci and were able to abort their seizures. He may be correct, but in my experience, if we include in our definition of mental imagery other internally prompted sensations, thoughts, and feelings, seizures originating in either hemisphere may be naturally arrested.

Which images are most effective? The image that uses the same channel as the aura may be the most effective. Odor counteracts odor; music counteracts music. But this theory seems to be only part of the truth. The man who goes fishing has a musical aura, but music plays no part in his fishing visualization. We do not use fear to block an aura of fear, but its opposite, the deep relaxation of bodily and emotional tension. Other individuals in the Pritchard research study used concentration and repeating a "prayer or poem to himself." "Going fishing," single-minded concentration, and meditating on a prayer or poem are all forms of deep relaxation. Four of these patients "showed significant changes in pulse rate, respiratory rate, and galvanic skin resistance."[15] These changes occur through deep relaxation. Other than those images that use the senses, the most effective ones will produce the neurophysiological effects of what Herbert Benson, M.D., has called the "relaxation response." Deep diaphragmatic breathing, in which you instruct your body to feel quiet and warm is the method of choice in my view.

When you practice blocking a seizure with any kind of mental image, make sure that you are in a safe place where you will not hurt yourself if you should fall or lose your balance. Sitting or lying down is best. Ask a member of your family or household or a support person to stay with you while you go through the initial trial experiments. Once you have established what works for you, see that it is effective, and gain confidence, you will be able to use this method anywhere, anytime, even on the concert stage as the woman who sniffed jasmine did.

If your aura is sensory, try a sensory response or a sensory image. If it begins with intense fear and anxiety, try the deep diaphragmatic breathing, the relaxation response. It shifts the body to a calm, relaxed mode. Try an angry "I won't let you do this to me!" Why this thought arrests a seizure is a mystery.

Commenting on psychical arrest, Wilder Penfield, M.D., writes that the important move seems to be that a patient "makes a voluntary mental effort to resist the first phase of the seizure."[16] This conscious mental effort may explain the effectiveness of the wide variety of mental images.

Using these methods of mental imagery to arrest seizures makes it possible to consider reducing medication. You need to have a consistent record of blocking your seizures. Any reduction in medication should be planned in consultation with your neurologist or physician. Remember that reducing or eliminating medication should be done slowly over an extended period of time.

In your notebook:

- Have you ever arrested a seizure? If you have, make note of what you did at what stage in the seizure's development. Tell your support person what you did so that he or she can remind you at the right moment, if that moment is observable to an outsider.
- Does your premonitory period or aura (not everyone has it) begin with a smell or a sound or a particular sensation or movement of some part of the body? The head turning away is common. Make note of this and share it with your support person.
- If it begins with a smell, buy a vial of concentrated essence of jasmine or peppermint at a pharmacy and keep it at hand. When you notice the odor typical of your seizure pattern, give yourself a strong whiff. The smell should be unpleasantly strong. Describe your experience with the above method.
- If your aura begins with a tingling sensation or movement in the arm or leg, ask someone to tie a tournequet firmly but not too tightly around the arm or leg above the line of march of the seizure. Then, if the tournequet does not arrest the seizure, that person can remove it before any numbness due to tightness sets in. Quick pricks with a pin (no need to draw blood) above the afflicted part have worked, too. Record your experience.
- Try movements of various kinds. Get up and move around. Walking should be done with a companion. Breathe deeply and slowly as you walk for an additional calming and relaxing effect. Are any of these effective for you? Make notes.
- If your aura begins with other sensations, experiment with the countering sensation that you think may work. Make note of what you try and what works for you. Tell your support person what it is so that he or she can help you remember to use it the next time.
- Practice mental imagery. Think of the happiest, most pleasurable, activity that you do. Sit quietly and comfortably, close your eyes, breathe deeply and slowly as you take yourself through a mental recreation of this happy experience. Feel all the sensations that accompany it: warm sun, cool breezes, the smells of woods and rivers and open fields, whatever. Be ready to imagine this experience again when you feel your aura. Make notes on your experience with this method.

Note: In this chapter we have used visualization and mental imagery as a specific method to arrest a seizure, but visualization is often practiced today in a broader context. Many people use it to rally and objectify the healing powers of the body and to help gain control of their bodies to fight many different kinds of illnesses. Dr. Bernard Siegel relates his use of mental imagery with cancer patients in his book, *Love, Medicine and Miracles* (Harper & Row, New York, 1986). In *Healing Yourself* by Martin L. Rossman, M.D. (Pocket Books, New York, 1987), there are detailed instructions for learning and using visualizations as well as the reasons why. If you wish to go further than seizure control using this method, you will find these two books instructive and inspiring.

21

Stopping Seizures with Another Person's Help

If seizures are viewed as the terminal link in a chain of behaviors, . . . [then] seizures can be prevented by interfering in preseizure behaviors.

—Steven Zlutnick et al.[1]

My husband told me that he could always tell when I was about to have a seizure because invariably I would turn to him with an odd expression on my face and say his name in a tone of voice that I never used at any other time. We think now that he could have made a move at just that moment that would have pulled me out of the seizure before it developed further, but we didn't know about seizure interventions until I read Dr. Robert Efron's articles years later.

I am not the only one who found Dr. Efron's work. Most of the research and literature on behavioral interventions have built on Robert Efron's study of the woman who sniffed jasmine. Since his articles appeared in the late 1950s, research activity on behavioral control of seizures has increased to the point where behavior psychologist David Mostofsky calls it an "explosion of writing" in the field. F. M. Forster published an influential paper in 1967. In 1973, R. B. Flannery and Joseph R. Cautela's "Seizures: Controlling the Uncontrollable" appeared, followed by R. G. Feldman and N. N. Paul's "Identity of Emotional Triggers in Epilepsy" in 1976. David Mostofsky's work with Barbara

Balaschak was published in 1977. Their compendium "Psychobiological Control of Seizures" brought together the behavioral techniques known to work in seizure intervention. The 1980s saw the publication of important British researchers like Peter Fenwick (1981), D. Chadwick and E. H. Reynolds (1985), and the Swedish work of Lennart Melin and P. Lessner with the American JoAnne Dahl.[2]

These developments in self-control of seizures rarely came and still rarely come to the attention of people with epilepsy. Exceptions are the practice of neurologist Joel Reiter and behavioral psychologist Donna Andrews in Santa Rosa, California. They work as a team in addressing the needs of the individual patient. There are others—Peter Fenwick and Laura Goldstein in London, Sarah Boden and Tim Betts in Birmingham, England, the staff of the epilepsy center Bethel in Bielefeld, Germany—but American epilepsy centers and practitioners tend to leave out behavioral interventions as part of the education and treatment of persons with epilepsy.

Behavior psychologists take the same view of the seizure sequence that neurologists do: that it entails the too-rapid firing of certain neurons and the progressive engagement of other neurons so that larger areas of the brain are involved. Where behavior psychologists differ is in the treatment. They see seizure as a sequence of behaviors. The timely use of a behavioral strategy will interrupt the sequence and abort the seizure.

How do you discover and learn an effective intervention strategy? Dr. JoAnne Dahl, an American working in Sweden, has emerged as a leading researcher in this field. She believes that a professional analysis is important, and she has developed a precise program for such analysis.[3] It follows the pattern of antecedents, behavior, and consequences sometimes called the "A-B-C's" of learned behavior.[4] In epilepsy the antecedents are the aura and/or triggering circumstances and conditions; the behavior is the seizure; and the consequences are the rewards and punishments (either internal or external) that reinforce seizure occurrence. In her work with both children and adults, Dr. Dahl has helped many individuals bring their seizures under control or eliminate them with behavioral methods. An eight-year follow-up[5] showed that the methods continued to work. Once a method has been learned and is recognized as successful, it can be used on your own. It is always with you.

In some ten years of experience in Swedish hospitals, Dr. Dahl has found that "arousal interventions" are most effective (see the previous chapter for sensory arousal and movement strategies). She stresses that seizures will not be alleviated if they are encouraged by some external response that rewards you for having a seizure. If you desire them for some internal reason, such as relief or excitement, you will limit your success.

Donna Andrews, Ph.D., the behavior psychologist who works with Joel Reiter, takes a similar approach. It is important to be systematic and to go step-by-step as you build your trust and confidence in these methods. Dr. Andrews draws on her own experience with seizures that have been under complete control without medication for some years. As a trained and experienced psychotherapist, she has successfully worked with patients who exhibit anger as part of their seizure pattern. She stresses the techniques that you can learn and use on your own.

Any method mentioned in the previous chapter can be learned and practiced with the help of a partner or support person. Also effective are the following two methods:

STARTLE-AND-SHAKE

A team of researchers from the University of Utah Medical School[6] set out to test the possibility of stopping seizures in a population of developmentally delayed schoolchildren. In almost every case the children had no more seizures.

The method the researchers used was startle-and-shake. It requires the existence of an observable preliminary behavior: staring at a flat surface, raising the arms, a strange tone of voice, hyperactivity, and so on. The support person acts to interrupt the sequence by following these steps:

1. Shout "No!" loudly and sharply to draw attention outward.

2. Grasp the person by the shoulders and shake him or her once. This changes the body's preseizure mode.

3. Give a little reward, a hug, an excited "You stopped it!" Offer any sort of praise or love for arresting the seizure. Let the good feeling, not candy or whatever, be the reward.

It is important with the startle-and-shake method to talk it over in advance. Let your support person know if this somewhat invasive method is acceptable to you. I have yet to hear of its failure in stopping a seizure.

THE SELF-CONTROL TRIAD

I am indebted to Joseph R. Cautela, Ph.D., a behavior psychologist, for bringing this method to my attention.[7] How does it work? When you feel your seizure begin:

1. Shout "No!" to yourself.

2. Then take a deep relaxing breath and do some relaxation exercises. See chapters 13, 14, and 15 for specific relaxation suggestions.

3. Finally, give yourself a reward by thinking of something very pleasant—fishing, being at the beach, eating your favorite ice cream, whatever.

Practice this method in advance of a seizure by imagining the preliminary signal and going through the steps. Do this in a safe environment where someone observes you and helps you to learn the sequence. Think of this method as an emergency prescription you take with you everywhere and at all times. You can fill it at a moment's notice.

The best thing about any of these methods is that by having fewer seizures, you are likely to have even fewer in the future. Anticonvulsant medication can be reduced if you and your doctor recognize your progress. With fewer seizures and lower dosages of medication, you gain a greater sense of control and alertness. Your life may approach normal for the first time.

In your notebook:

- Has an external act ever interrupted a seizure for you? What was it?
- How can you turn that occurrence into a systematic action that your support person can implement? Try it. Describe what happened.
- Discuss the startle-and-shake procedure with a support person and be ready to have that person act when he or she sees your typical preliminary behavior.
- Did the procedure work in stopping a seizure or in blocking aspects of it? Make notes of what happened.

22

Learning Biofeedback

Joel Reiter, M.D.

Biofeedback as a widely recognized discipline is barely a teenager. But in its short life it has been documented in some ten thousand professional articles and its practitioners and scientists number in the many thousands around the world.

—John Basmajian, M.D.[1]

Biofeedback is as American as apple pie. As a nation we love our cars, VCRs, and computers. This love of technology has spawned biofeedback, a method of using a machine to tell us the state of our bodies. One particular form of biofeedback—EEG biofeedback—is an especially useful tool for people with epilepsy.

In our daily lives, we are subjected to constant stimulation. Driving to work can be a life-threatening experience; we must look at the road ahead, the rear-view mirror, and to either side. Walking on a city sidewalk or crossing a street demands the same level of vigilance. Even if our own homes are peaceful, newspapers and television subject us to a constant barrage of catastrophes, which results in most of us being overaroused a good deal of the time, with our brain waves in an alert (beta) state.

In other chapters of this book, Adrienne Richard has taught you deep diaphragmatic breathing, progressive relaxation, and meditation skills. If you practice one of these methods daily, there is a good chance that you will be in an awake and relaxed (alpha) state more of the time. Adrienne and I have heard from many people that these techniques,

when practiced regularly, lead to marked reduction in seizures. Dr. Steve Whitman and his colleagues at Northwestern University recently found that people with uncontrolled
seizures can reduce the frequency of their seizures by about
50 percent if they perform daily progressive relaxation exercises.[2] This study supports other studies mentioned by
Adrienne in previous chapters.

However, it is one thing to practice meditation, deep
breathing, or progressive relaxation every day and another
to achieve the desired result—an awake and relaxed state. I
became aware of this difficulty when a young doctor asked
me to see his wife, Alice, who was having constant headaches. I diagnosed muscle contraction headaches, also
called tension headaches. I thought Alice's treatment would
be simple since she was already experienced in meditation.
She had stopped meditating because her life became too
busy. I suggested that she resume daily meditation. To my
dismay, her headaches were not relieved at all!

At the time I had a biofeedback machine in my office
that could measure both muscle tension and EEG. I decided
to use it to try to find an explanation for Alice's experience.
I hooked her up to the biofeedback equipment and asked
her to practice meditation in her usual way. Then I asked
her to tell me when she was in a relaxed state. Surprisingly,
the EEG biofeedback machine showed that she was still in
an alert, or beta, state. When she stopped meditating, she
went into a drowsing theta state. But she never went into an
awake and relaxed alpha state. Thus, she performed meditation as she lived the rest of her life: with pressure and
tension. She wasn't able to relax enough to achieve the
desired result of meditation, which is the awake and relaxed
alpha state. No wonder meditation hadn't helped her headaches.

I next asked Alice to let go of her concern about the
result as she meditated. I told her that the EEG biofeedback
machine would let her know if she was in an awake and
relaxed state. Nothing changed until one day she said, "I
don't give a damn what happens; I'm just going to meditate
for the fun of it." After that, the EEG biofeedback machine

began to register increased alpha activity. Alice achieved the desired result of meditation and stopped having headaches.

Alice's experience and others like it showed me how hard it can be for many patients to let down enough to allow meditation, breathing exercises, or progressive relaxation exercises to really work for them. The work ethic teaches Americans how to get things done, not how to relax. Even our recreational activities tend to be goal-oriented and stimulating, rather than allowing us to relax.

On the other hand, we Americans are comfortable using machines in work and at play. I wondered whether an EEG biofeedback machine could help other patients, particularly those who had uncontrolled seizures, achieve better results from these techniques.

What is EEG biofeedback? Is there any scientific basis for it, or is it just the latest hocus-pocus? To answer these questions I will review the research that led to the development of modern-day biofeedback equipment. The story begins in 1929 when Dr. Walter Cannon described the relationship between the autonomic or involuntary nervous system and the emotions. In his classic book, *Bodily Changes in Pain, Hunger, Fear and Rage*, the famous Harvard physiologist described the ways in which the autonomic or involuntary nervous system regulates blood pressure, heart rate, gastrointestinal motility, blood vessel tone, and other basic bodily functions to keep them within normal range. He demonstrated that physical, psychological, and emotional stress stimulates the autonomic nervous system to speed up the heart, raise the blood pressure, increase stomach acid, and make a person feel jazzed up. Dr. Cannon pointed out that "not only were there visible manifestations of the expression of emotions, there were also internal correlates that cannot be seen and, indeed, are not even felt."[3]

If you are crossing the street and a truck comes at you, it is appropriate for you to run. In order to run fast, your heart rate picks up and your blood pressure increases. If you keep imagining that the truck is going to hit you, your autonomic nervous system will keep your heart racing and your stomach churning even though the threat is no longer physically present. The mere psychological perception of threat can trigger the same autonomic nervous system overarousal that occurs when you are actually confronted with a physical threat. The sense of being out of control that we call *anxiety* is associated with this type of autonomic system overarousal.

The autonomic nervous system is also known as the involuntary nervous system because it works without your having to think about it. For thirty years after Dr. Cannon's classic research, it was medical dogma that individuals could not voluntarily control their autonomic nervous system activity. Then in the 1960s, experimental psychologist Neal Miller taught rats to control their heart rate and blood pressure. If rats could learn to control their autonomic nervous system, what could people learn to do? Happily, clinical researchers found that people were able to learn to change their heart rate, hand temperature, or blood pressure. This learning was based on a conditioning model in which a person is given a reward for completing a task. For example, if the task is to decrease blood pressure, each time a person lowers his blood pressure a certain number of points he receives a quarter. By repeating this task successfully many times the person learns to lower his blood pressure at will.

The next step in teaching people to control their autonomic nervous systems was to develop electronic equipment that could measure specific physiologic responses controlled by the autonomic nervous system. Not only could it measure blood pressure, hand temperature, tightness of muscles, heart rate, or brain waves but the equipment could also give a sound (auditory) or light (visual) signal to let a person know when he had reached his goal. This equipment, called biofeedback equipment, gave rise to the new field of biofeedback therapy. Dr. John Basmajian, a founding father of this new form of treatment, defines biofeedback as "the technique of using equipment (usually electronic) to reveal to human beings some of their internal physiologic events, normal and abnormal, in the form of visual and auditory signals in order to teach them to manipulate these otherwise involuntary or unfelt events by manipulating the displayed signals. This technique inserts a person's volition into the gap of an open feedback loop—hence the artificial name biofeedback—here necessarily a human being must want to voluntarily change the signals because they meet some goals."[4]

The type of biofeedback machine that will help you depends on your symptoms. For example, a muscle biofeedback instrument helps people with muscle contraction headaches, a temperature machine helps those with migraine, and an EEG biofeedback machine helps those with seizures. To do EEG biofeedback, electrodes are attached to a person's scalp. The electrodes are hooked up to an EEG biofeedback machine that measures brain waves—the difference in electrical potential between the electrodes. EEG biofeedback equipment is designed to make a soft noise when you go into a particular brain wave state. When the noise is present you are in that particular brain wave. Your doctor or biofeedback therapist may suggest that you would have better control over your seizures if you learn to go into a particular brain wave state more of the time.

In Part II, chapter 3, I described how your brain waves change between waking and sleeping, relaxation and alertness, seizure activity and no seizure activity. For example, if you are awake and relaxed you are in the alpha state of 8 to 12 cycles per second. While you are concentrating to understand this chapter you are in the beta state of 13 to 30 cycles per second. If this chapter fails to grab your interest, you will go into the drowsing theta state of 4 to 7 cycles per second. Finally, if I were to succeed in boring you completely, you might go to sleep and be in the delta state of 1 to 4 cycles per second.

Is there any brain wave state you can go into to decrease the likelihood of having a seizure? My experience with patients and the research of psychologists M. B. Sterman and Joel Lubar indicate that different brain waves states are beneficial for different people with seizures. This finding should not come as a surprise if you have been impressed by Adrienne Richard's description of the different things people do to increase control over their seizures. For example, she described her own success using meditation and progressive relaxation exercises that most likely put her into an alpha brain wave state. The startle-and-shake routine she described probably increases awake and alert, or beta, brain wave activity.

My clinical research has focused on helping people with complex partial epilepsy improve control over their seizures. Only 50 percent of individuals with complex partial epilepsy have total control over their seizures using anticonvulsant medications. Years ago, I was struck by the EEG pattern of many of my patients with complex partial epilepsy. Their routine EEGs showed an overabundance of the theta brain wave state normally seen in drowsiness. Many had no background alpha activity. I thought they might achieve better control over seizures if they could learn to go into a normal awake and relaxed alpha state at will. Donna Andrews and I developed an EEG biofeedback training technique for people with complex partial seizures.

If you had complex partial seizures and came to see me, I would order a routine diagnostic EEG. From this EEG, Donna Andrews and I could discover which frontotemporal brain area shows the slowest or most abnormal brain wave activity. We would then teach you deep breathing, progressive relaxation, and imagery skills. Learning these exercises would allow you to increase alpha activity over that abnormal area, while decreasing slow theta brain wave activity. Once you learned to reliably produce alpha activity at an amplitude of greater than 50 microvolts, the frequency of your complex partial seizures would most likely decrease dramatically.

There is nothing magical about going into an alpha brain wave state in order to decrease seizures. In fact, other researchers have trained people to increase brain wave states other than alpha to improve control over seizures. However, all of the methods have a common denominator: They decrease slower theta brain wave activity. If reading about EEG biofeedback has heightened your interest, you may want to read the excellent review articles by Dr. M. B. Sterman and Dr. Joel Lubar referenced later in this book. Detailed instructions about the use of EEG biofeedback are available in my book, *Taking Control of Your Epilepsy: A Workbook for Patients and Professionals*.

Suppose you have success in reducing your seizures through EEG biofeedback training. Will you have to carry a biofeedback machine around with you? Obviously not! The techniques you use to learn to control your brain waves—including deep breathing, progressive relaxation, and meditation—are the same methods that Adrienne Richard has described in other chapters. EEG biofeedback training lets you know that the exercises are working for you. It is as if your body and brain say, "Aha, now we know what it feels like to be in that brain wave state!" As soon as you know that you are doing the exercises in an effective way, you won't need a biofeedback machine anymore. But you will have to keep doing your exercises!

PART SEVEN

TAKING ACTION

23

Designing Your
Personal Program

*Illness needs to be viewed within the context of the entire
life . . . of the patient. Identical disorders need to be
considered quite differently in view of the person. . . .
Patients can and do emerge from psychological and physical disorders with increased rather than impaired functioning.*

—Kenneth R. Pelletier[1]

Epilepsy is often referred to in the medical literature
as "the epilepsies" because of the variety of seizure manifestations. Add to this variety the individual differences among
people who experience epilepsy, and an almost bewildering
array of seizure patterns emerges. One person's pattern may
differ significantly from another's, although both people
"have epilepsy," and may even have the same general type
of seizure. "Identical disorders," as Dr. Pelletier comments,
"need to be considered quite differently in view of the
person." This statement cannot be truer than it is for epilepsy. When it comes to designing a self-care program for
yourself, you need to keep this fact in mind. Your program
must be custom-designed for you.

Each element in this book is important in an effective
and ongoing self-care program. Each one contributes to
emerging from the onset or longtime experience of epilepsy
"with increased rather than impaired functioning."

Read over the notes you have taken after each chapter,
starting at the beginning of the book and going to the end.

Use your notebook to make additional notes and comments about the following:

Your own story. From your account of your first seizure, or the first one you remember in detail, what stands out for you today? Do you have any intuitions about what may be helpful for you in caring for yourself that arise as you reread your account? In mulling over her own seizures, the epilepsy counselor Donna Andrews found herself asking, Why do I not have seizures all the time when I have seizure spikes on my EEG all the time? The question proved to be the key to her recovery.

The social and cultural milieu around you. Your seizures do not occur in a vacuum but within a family or a social context where certain convictions and values are strongly held, and within a community and a culture with certain values and convictions. Only a portion of these beliefs will be consciously held, making them all the more powerful. Epilepsy has a peculiar ability to arouse deeply held fears and taboos. It may also indicate the potential for transcendent experience.

What cultural convictions about epilepsy have increased or decreased your suffering? What are your own convictions and beliefs about epilepsy? How do these help you in coming to your own terms with it? How can you behave in order to minimize the negatives and maximize the positives?

Information about epilepsy. Are you well informed about epilepsy? Dr. Joel Reiter's chapters are a wonderfully rich presentation of what is currently known. The neurosciences are the most rapidly growing area of medicine today, and more and more will emerge in the future.

Make note of what was of particular interest to you and your case in those chapters. Keep your eye out for more in these areas. Ask the Epilepsy Foundation of America to put your name on their mailing list for the periodic update of publications on epilepsy.

Diagnosis and treatment. Do you know exactly what kind of seizures your physician or neurologist thinks you have? Precise knowledge can be helpful and reassuring.

Does this diagnosis fit what you experience? Some diagnoses may be incorrect. One woman writes to me that she diagnosed herself from a newspaper account of "Geschwind's Syndrome," asked to have her medication changed accordingly, and achieved better control, although she is still not persuaded that the diagnosis is entirely correct and helpful.

The diagnosis determines treatment, particularly medication and dosage. How does your system respond to the drug or drugs that have been prescribed for you? Are your seizures controlled? They will be in some 50 or 60 percent of cases, depending on the type of seizure. Does the medication exhibit side effects? These can be nonexistent, to mild and tolerable, to debilitating and even life-threatening. A change in medication may make a total difference, and it may simply make matters worse. You must observe yourself. Make notes. Report your experience to your doctor.

Today monotherapy (use of only one drug) is recommended. Many people are on two or more. Ask your physician about changing to a one-drug therapy.

If you wish to go without medication, also consult your doctor. If you have been on anticonvulsants, this change should be done very gradually. If you are a woman considering pregnancy, or a person who has gone two years or more without a seizure, or if you have religious or personal objections to medication, or if you find your seizures enriching in some way, going without medication should be seriously considered with your neurologist.

Your personal self-care program. Your attitude toward yourself, your observation of yourself, adopting preventive measures, and using effective interventions are the four pillars of epilepsy self-care. Medication cannot be expected to do everything for you.

ATTITUDE

Some of you may have noticed that I have tried in this book not to use the word *epileptic* as a noun, with good reason. To my mind, and to many neurologists as well, the word *epileptic* carries the connotation of defining the whole person in terms of one part of that person. A person with epileptic seizures is many things and has many aspects and facets that he or she lives out, and the affliction of seizures is a part of this life but not the only part, not the defining part. This attitude of being a person with seizures, not an epileptic, is an essential ingredient in gaining some control over this condition.

How is it possible to maintain the daily self-care practices and still not think of yourself as an epileptic? Self-care for seizures is no more difficult than maintaining any daily health and hygiene routines. They become habitual and take very little conscious decision making to practice.

More important, a sense of your own wholeness that is larger and greater than the sum of its parts underlies everything. In the workshops that I give I often take people through a process of visualizing this wholeness:

1. Sit comfortably with your eyes closed and do a few relaxation exercises in your chair: the neck rolls on page 147, and the short form of progressive relaxation on page 145. Breathe slowly and deeply as you do so.

2. When you feel relaxed, visualize a small person just outside beyond your closed eyes. Let that person enter your head through the space between the eyebrows.

3. Now take that person through your entire body, visiting all the healthy places: the heart, the stomach, the liver, and so on. Stop briefly at any unhealthy ones: the sore shoulder, blocked bowel, knot of anxiety, or whatever.

4. In the end bring the person to the head again and visit that part of the brain—temporal lobe or deeper areas—that is involved in your seizures. Imagine this person soothing that part, or massaging it gently, helping it to relax and feel better, to function more normally.

5. Allow the little person to leave the way he or she came in. Breathe deeply for a few minutes and open your eyes. In your notebook write or draw a picture of what has occurred. The end result of this exercise is often a sense of general good feeling and body unity, a rallying of helpful forces around the problem area.

At the close of a workshop we usually go through the mini-series of progressive relaxation exercises, close our eyes, and do the deep diaphragmatic breathing. Once we are deeply relaxed, I suggest the following affirmations. Just repeat to yourself:

> I need my brain to live.
> I want my brain to function calmly and normally.
> I will do everything I can to help my brain to function calmly and normally.

Repeating this affirmation at the deepest point during the practice of the relaxation exercises and again just before sleep has remarkably helpful effects.

These exercises in combination convey a sense and a mental image of our being larger and greater in our totality than the disorder that is only one part of us.

OBSERVATION

You must observe your physical and emotional responses closely to learn what conditions and circumstances make you seizure-prone. Every time a seizure breaks through, ask yourself:

> Did I take my medication?
> Was I under emotional stress? What were the reasons for the stress? For example, work, relationships, placing unreasonable demands on yourself.
> Was I under physical stress? Fatigue, illness, menstruation, constipation, too much sun.
> Have I maintained my exercise program?
> What about my diet? Alcohol, excessive caffeine, sweets, in particular.

Observing the aura that may precede a seizure is the most important observation of all. Make note of what your aura feels like and tell yourself what you are going to do when you feel it. If you don't observe an aura, others around you may. Work with that other person in preparation for your aura's occurrence.

Auras may be strange experiences: feeling "spacey" and/or light-headed; detecting nonexistent smells, sights, and sounds; hearing voices; "surges" of feeling through the neck and head; feeling nervous and jumpy; increased intuitive powers and mystical religious experiences; and many other unusual sensations and feelings such as inexplicable mood swings and irritability. During this period of high risk you need to take care of yourself—get enough rest, eat properly, release tension, and avoid emotional and physical stressors until the period passes and you are back to normal.

PREVENTION

Life-style, stress, tension, exercise, diet, and environmental hazards are the areas where change or modification may be indicated for you.

1. Go over your personal notes at the end of each chapter in Part V to know what is or is not helpful for you.
2. Make a daily schedule for practicing the exercises that help you.
3. Include in this daily routine

a. Some gentle exercise
b. Some form of physical relaxation: progressive muscle relaxation, or another form of gentle stretches
c. Deep diaphragmatic breathing or another form of breathing exercise

4. Make changes in diet, if needed, for a balanced high-fiber, low-fat, moderate-protein, low-sugar diet. Include a multivitamin with B_6 and B_{12} and minerals. You may need supplemental calcium and vitamin D because their uptake into the body is inhibited by anticonvulsant medication.

Notice if you feel better, more energized, more alert, more buoyant in spirit. Give yourself time—three to six months or more to evaluate this. A self-care program is not as immediately effective as swallowing medication may be.

INTERVENTIONS

Know your seizure pattern or patterns and the aura that may precede them. Be aware of what interventions you or another person can make. Talk about these in advance to be ready to act. Practice them so that you are familiar with the procedure. If an intervention involves an act by another person, be sure that the other person has your permission to do whatever is needed, for example, take you by the shoulders and give you a shake and/or shout your name.

Keep track of your seizures: their type, frequency, and intensity. Do they diminish? Do they change? Do you have a clear idea or a sense of what you are doing that is most effective as a preventive or interventive method? Keep that in mind as the basis for action.

Once you have created your program, it must be practiced, daily at first, always several times a week. "Homework is absolutely essential," writes Dennis Jaffe, Ph.D., in *Healing from Within*. "The goal [emphasis mine] is to increase your awareness of when your body is functioning improperly, and enhance your ability to immediately reverse an inappropriate or ineffective psychophysiological response."[2]

Some people find that maintaining their own self-care programs is difficult. Support from others around you in daily home and work life is enormously important. Support groups can be helpful as well.

A CHECKLIST FOR MANAGING YOUR LIFE-STYLE FOR BETTER HEALTH AND GREATER SEIZURE CONTROL

1. Let stress and tension go from the muscles by practicing progressive muscle relaxation and other gentle exercises, and from the neck and shoulders by doing neck rolls, shoulder shrugs, and "the chicken wing."

2. Achieve deeper levels of relaxation through practicing deep diaphragmatic breathing twenty minutes or more each day.

3. Improve general health through a high-fiber, low-fat, low-sugar, moderate-protein diet and gentle exercise.

4. Increase energy and alertness with a daily multiple vitamin plus a minerals supplement that includes vitamins B_6, B_{12}, folic acid, manganese, and magnesium, and with additional daily calcium—calcium carbonate is preferred.

5. Avoid certain substances such as alcohol, caffeine, sugars, sweeteners, nicotine, hard drugs, pesticides, and heavy metals.

6. Use interventions to block seizures. Dispel fear and anxiety through the deep diaphragmatic breathing. Ask an observer to use the startle-and-shake procedure. Find your own personal methods of mental imagery.

7. Take good care of yourself during periods of high risk for seizures by following (1) through (5) above.

24

Negotiating the World

Though the general public is more enlightened about epilepsy today, the myth dies hard.

—Richard Pollak[1]

The myths about epilepsy—that a person is in some way incompetent, functionally compromised, or close to crazy—are dying, but their death is slow. As a consequence, people with epilepsy face some problems of living in the world that others with long-term or chronic health problems do not face. There are the personal and interpersonal considerations discussed in the course of this book, but there are other issues as well. The diagnosis of epilepsy puts you in possible conflict with the law. There is the problem of obtaining or keeping a driver's license. Coverage by health and life insurance may be difficult to obtain. Access to state and federal services for the handicapped is problematic. Jobs may be hard to get and harder to hold. Each time a criminal case reaches court where the defense is based on the defendant's epilepsy, the accompanying publicity means another round of social and psychological setbacks for everyone with epilepsy.

The situation is much better than it used to be just a few decades ago. Colonies for persons with epilepsy were common into the 1920s, although epilepsy was known not to be contagious well before that. In some states laws preventing people with epilepsy from marrying remained on the books into the 1950s, and taboos against marriage persist in other parts of the world. The American immigration laws prevented anyone with epilepsy from entering the country even for medical treatment until the most recent revisions. The stresses that people with seizures endure in getting jobs and on the job, in their private lives and relationships, and in living with a terrible secret testify to this society's residue of superstition. In every workshop that I have given for people with seizures, there has been at least one person, usually a woman, who has spent a long period in a psychiatric hospital incorrectly diagnosed as "mental." Much work needs to be done still to improve our lives.

DRIVING

The one issue that confronts every person with epilepsy is the question of being a licensed driver. Every state Department of Motor Vehicles regulates under what conditions that person will be licensed, and there are fifty different versions that range from mild and reasonable to highly restrictive (until recently, California). The toughest part of regulations is the seizure-free period required before a license is obtainable. As of 1990,[2] twenty-seven states required a year-long seizure-free period. A few of those states modify this rule for certain kinds of seizures and/or a doctor's recommendation. Only ten states do not require a seizure-free period. All but three states make keeping that license dependent on a periodic physician's report. Seven states demand that doctors report any patients with seizures, a restriction that affects doctor–patient confidentiality and inhibits some people with seizures from getting the help they need. In addition, the physician may fear liability as a third party and will obey the letter of his or her state's law.

Are persons with epilepsy a real threat on the highway? No more so than drivers with other medical conditions, according to Julian Waller, M.D., an epidemiologist and highway safety expert at the University of Vermont School of Medicine. "Drivers with chronic illnesses," Dr. Waller told me, "have about twice as many crashes per million miles driven as drivers the same age and sex without these problems. But only one-fourth of the increase can be attributed to obvious clinical episodes." Dr. Waller says that people with epilepsy do not account for more accidents per capita than teenagers, not a group with the best record in the world but nonetheless licensed without much question. The National Safety Council[3] reported that in 1977 only "one in 10,000 traffic accidents appear to be related to seizures" and that these accidents "tended not to be as serious as other accidents." The council's most recent update concludes, "Accidents caused by seizures involve the driver's vehicle alone or an immovable object 80 percent of the time and tend to occur in less populated and developed areas." Nevertheless, the occasional accident where there are fatalities always makes headlines and obscures the general rule.

Despite these findings, the licenses of persons with epilepsy are revoked more often than any other group except drug users with a history of prior arrest! No wonder that those of us with epilepsy feel that society punishes us unfairly. The social, economic, and personal consequences of being without a driver's license are enormous. Driving to get to a job, or to run a household, particularly in parts of the country where mass transportation is virtually nonexistent, becomes difficult and expensive. Teenagers are deprived of their major rite of passage into adulthood when they cannot obtain a driver's license, and adults are deprived of the principal method of identification.

Licensing laws for passenger cars, Dr. Waller comments, "need to balance concern for the individual and concern for the public. The point is not to try to prevent all crashes." The laws, he emphasizes, should be based on established data, taking into account seizure type and frequency. For example, seizures that occur only during sleep, the so-called nocturnal seizure, should not prevent a person from getting a driver's license, nor should seizures that do not affect consciousness or motor coordination. The Wisconsin law puts some responsibility on the individual to monitor his own condition. He must be aware of the effects of stress on lapses of consciousness and the need to be regular with prescribed medications.

In addition, I believe, the laws must also permit physicians to exercise their best judgment on behalf of their patients without undue liability. And they must not undermine doctor–patient confidentiality. Some people will hesitate to seek the help they need and will simply lie on the driver's license application.

Even a licensed driver with epilepsy needs to drive carefully and thoughtfully. Here are some rules for playing it safe:

Leave the driving to others whenever possible.
Drive a car with a stick shift for greater control and alertness on your part. Never use cruise control.
Drive defensively, safely, and at reasonable speeds.
Keep children in the back seat, safety belts buckled.
Pull off the road immediately if you feel odd.
Don't drive when you feel at risk (e.g., fatigued, ill, under great stress).
Avoid driving in heavy traffic, at night, or in poor weather.
Avoid conditions such as flickering lights and blurred visibility that may provoke trance states.

INSURANCE

Coverage by insurance companies varies enormously, and the clauses in employee–employer contracts that pertain to epilepsy differ from contract to contract. The differences are too great to cover here. Suffice it to say, life and health insurance have been denied to persons with epilepsy. It is necessary to become an advocate for what you need. The book, *Children with Epilepsy*,[4] is excellent for its delineation of the process for becoming an effective advocate for your rights or the rights of others. The Epilepsy Foundation of America is investigating this problem as well.

GOVERNMENT SERVICES

Most states and the federal government provide financial

aid and/or support services for persons with disabilities. Often these are defined as developmental disabilities that have begun prior to the age of twenty-one. Some 25 percent of all cases of epilepsy begin after age twenty-one, and if this is so for you, you may be denied access to services or financial assistance. Other provisions may be specifically for the handicapped, and epilepsy may or may not be included in your state's definition of a handicap. Again it is necessary to become an advocate. Reach your state and congressional representatives and find out what you need to do to be an effective spokesperson for yourself and for others.

If you have a local epilepsy association, you may be able to join with others with similar concerns. Advocacy in groups tends to be more effective than individually. Again, consult the book, *Children with Epilepsy*, for solid assistance.

EDUCATION

Antidiscrimination laws specify that a person cannot be fired or denied access to education on the grounds of a disability. In recent years, both Rutgers, the New Jersey state university, and Swarthmore College, a distinguished private school, have acted to deny admittance to individuals with epilepsy. In each case the individual fought against the ruling and won.

WORK

Cases of job discrimination have been so numerous in the past that a special program for persons with epilepsy was established by the U.S. Department of Labor and the Epilepsy Foundation of America in 1976. The study that preceded the program had shown that "epilepsy ranked the lowest of all handicaps from which employers were willing to employ" and that "only 2 percent of persons with epilepsy were served by state vocational rehabilitation programs."[5] The Training and Placement Services—TAPS programs—were and are continuing to be set up to meet the obvious and critical need. They are available in many cities around the country.

A TAPS workshop teaches the effective tools in getting a job: how to write a résumé, cover letter, and thank-you letter; how to set up an interview and learn interview skills; how to present yourself on the telephone. Most important are the self-esteem and motivation the job applicant acquires in the course of the workshop.

An employment specialist told me, "Disclosure is the hardest thing we deal with. Learning how to advocate for yourself, to say in a nonthreatening manner that you have epilepsy, deciding when to disclose and when not to disclose—[these] are the most difficult skills and issues we deal with."

CRIMINAL ACCUSATIONS

Because certain seizure types are characterized by automatic behavior with total amnesia afterward, epilepsy is often in the news. The crimes may be minor—shoplifting and the like; or they may be major—murder and violence.

The most famous recent case is that of Jack Ruby, who shot Harvey Oswald—the man accused of assassinating President John F. Kennedy—when Ruby accosted Oswald in the basement of the Dallas police station. In Ruby's trial for murder his defense attorneys claimed that he had committed this act unconsciously during an epileptic seizure. In another instance, reported on the recent television series, "The Mind" (PBS, 1988), a woman with epilepsy commits violent acts but has no such occurrences after the brain surgery that eliminated her epilepsy. The painter, Vincent van Gogh, was arrested and jailed after the incident when he slashed his ear lobe and probably an artery. Some eighty persons petitioned the mayor of Arles to have van Gogh confined. He wrote his brother Theo, "I had inflicted a wound on myself, I had done nothing of the sort to them."[6]

Nonetheless, he was confined to a mental institution for a year.

The journalist, Richard Pollak, himself a person with epilepsy, has researched much of the material on criminal cases where epilepsy is part of the explanation of a crime's occurrence.[7] In the case of Jack Ruby, the epilepsy argument was destroyed by the prosecution on the basis that premeditation was obvious in Ruby's act. It was pointed out that the characteristic impulsiveness and disorganization of such an act, if it should be caused by epilepsy, was absent. In conclusion, Pollak believes that violent crimes due to epilepsy are rare indeed. Corroborating this conclusion is the research on inmates at an Illinois prison. It shows no greater an incidence of epilepsy among prisoners than in the general population outside prison. Other researchers, however, find that epilepsy is "two or four times more prevalent . . . but socioeconomic status may be a factor."[8] Richard Pollak writes:

> Few neurologists rule out the possibility that in extremely rare instances epilepsy *might* [italics his] play some role in violent criminal behavior. As yet, however, no scientific proof supports the contention that epileptics can commit goal-directed, aggressive crimes during seizures.[9]

The amnesia characteristic of many seizures has served a useful function in the fictional crime literature of seizure. Richard Pollak in his suspense novel, *The Episode*,[10] has the murder weapon planted in the journalist/hero's laundry during his epileptic episode that gives the book its title. The hero has no remembrance of that period of time and becomes a sleuth to defend himself. The criminal charges that are brought against the linen weaver, Silas Marner,[11] stem from a similar episode of which Marner has no memory, and he is cast out of his community because of it.

The drama and dilemmas of epilepsy make great fiction created either by writers or defense lawyers "scrambling for a dramatic plea." This literature can complicate life even further for persons who live with epilepsy, even as it illuminates and fascinates as literature.

The life of a person with epilepsy is full of pitfalls (no pun intended). There are not only the seizures themselves and the complex psychological stresses they engender but the social and political reactions from the world around us as well. Their persistence in dying hard raises the real dilemma of when, if ever, to be open about your epilepsy. Living with a dreaded secret does not make for good psychological health, but coming out in the open runs the risk of activating the latent taboos that continue to lie beneath the surface with many people. Even your doctor may have latent prejudices. One woman told me that her neurologist accuses her of "interictal personality problems" whenever she disagrees with him or challenges his judgment. Through this kind of bullying the neurologist reveals more of himself than he does of his patient. It is an example of the subtle use of epilepsy against the person. As a consequence, revealing yourself as someone with seizures remains a serious question.

No one is required to do so, and the right to privacy protects us from being forced. However, that right is often threatened. In an op-ed article in the *New York Times*, Richard Pollak[12] writes that mandatory drug testing will expose persons with epilepsy who take phenobarbital and make it necessary for them to come out in the open whether they wish to or not.

I went for over twenty years without telling my sons about my epilepsy. The medication gave me complete control. I didn't have to tell them, and I didn't. When my sons were in their early twenties—I was diagnosed when I was pregnant with my second son!—I broke the news very casually one afternoon. My eldest son was outraged. "Why didn't you tell us?" he exclaimed.

"I didn't have to," I said. "Why should I?"

"But we might have had to take care of you," he said.

I was stunned. They wanted to take care of me! I thought of myself as the mother, the one who took care of them, an extension of myself as the competent person in the world who can take care of herself, on top of everything. I would have had to let go of some of that to share my secret with them. Would it have harmed them to take care of me from time to time? Of course not, quite the opposite. It would have been developmental for them and for me, as well.

At a recent meeting of the epilepsy association, where I sit on the board of directors, we discussed the composition of the board and the question of what percentage should be people with epilepsy. Some members such as myself have a history of seizures, but no one knows for sure about many others, because disclosure is not and cannot be required. It seemed to me that if we do not feel safe enough to acknowledge our epilepsy in such a group, the group is functioning poorly. But the larger picture is obvious. Many persons do not choose to expose themselves even in the safest and most accepting surroundings.

There is no easy answer to whether you should or should not disclose your epilepsy. The bitter joke among people with seizures is that the only ones who disclose are those who have to. Their seizures are not controlled. For mental health and social ease it is obviously best to be open about epilepsy, but your decision to do so must take into account your personal situation.

In your notebook:

- How do you feel about letting the world or some portion of it know about your epilepsy?
- What consequence do you believe revealing it will have?
- Consider revealing your condition to a selected few in a circle wider than those who now know and show acceptance. Listen for feelings and attitudes. Find ways to counter negative positions with factual information. Many people are simply frightened and don't know what to do. When they learn that the most helpful thing is to do nothing but see that you don't hurt yourself in falling, they relax and accept the possibility that you may have a seizure.

PART EIGHT

CLOSING THOUGHTS

25

"Portals"

*A wellness can be genuine even if caused by an illness.
And such a paradoxical wellness may even confer a lasting
benefit.*

—Oliver Sacks, M.D.[1]

The most remarkable aspect of epilepsy to me is its
capacity to bridge the gulf between mind and brain and
body. A seizure is an event that occurs in the brain and its
effects are noticed in the brain and body. The mind, each
individual's complex collection of awareness, attitudes, and
abilities, is also dependent on the brain, but it can be
brought to bear on these events of the brain, altering frequency and intensity and even the kind of seizure.

In thinking about the effect of the mind on seizures I find
myself pondering the fact that all the diverse methods described in this book help some persons under some conditions to attain greater or complete seizure control. A course
of medications taken regularly helps many. Changing their
diet helps some people, while a regimen of special nutrients
helps others. Getting rid of stress and keeping the body as
relaxed as possible helps still others, while a combination
of strategies relieves another group. Interventions, either
self-imposed or done by others, are an effective method for
many. These diverse experiences make me wonder what
helping power is invested in these methods. Does a common
denominator exist among them?

Is there a self-control center in the brain that is activated
whenever we undertake a self-help program? Does a self-
care regimen by its very nature reset the homeostatic
mechanisms deep in the brain so that they operate in

accordance with the new plan? These mechanisms are often compared to the thermostat of a furnace. Once we set it at 68 degrees, the furnace acts accordingly. Once we set our brains for self-care, do they then function in the appropriate manner?

Does a sense of self-control give us a detachment that emphasizes our wellness and deemphasizes this affliction, and as a consequence do its eruptions and disruptions diminish? Does each one of these strategies stimulate the release of or synthesis of certain biochemicals that calm the neurons? Do we awaken an "inner healer" or Dr. Albert Schweitzer's "doctor inside"? Perhaps a willingness to take control of our own condition is just that.

Do we shift our emotional commitment from the benefits of illness to the benefits of wellness?

Is any one of these strategies simply making the mental effort that Wilder Penfield noticed as effective in "psychical arrest"?

I do not know the answers to these questions. Not long ago I visualized seizure activity in my brain. That is, I thought about it and allowed a mental image to arise. The image that materialized was one of little men in electric blue bodysuits dancing about, shooting sparks. I asked them what they were doing, and they replied, "Oh, just fooling around, having fun." I told them I'd rather they didn't do that in my head. At first they continued what they were doing, but gradually they quieted, sat down, and looked resigned. I was reminded of hyperactive children who can't stop until they are given firm but loving direction. I can see my little granddaughter's resigned expression when her father says to her, "I love you unconditionally, but in five minutes you are going to bed." She knows she is loved and she knows she is going to bed. Can control of a seizure work in a similar manner? The cerebral traffic controller, that is, the mind, says to the hyperactive neurons, gently but firmly, "I can't have you doing that." And so they don't.

As remarkable as its bridging of the mind/body dichotomy is epilepsy's power to stimulate thought. A seizure is "just a seizure" without great meaning in and of itself. Its meaning lies in what it makes us think of, in how we interpret it. Over the centuries and across cultural lines seizures have evoked notably similar responses as *morbus deificus* and *morbus demoniacus*, the disease of the gods and the disease of the devil, a valued gift or a hideous curse.

The most plausible explanation, for me, of this persistent and near-universal interpretation lies in a seizure's resemblance to death. The sudden attack has no visible cause—no blood, no wound, no pain. Consciousness is suddenly lost or attention suddenly absent. Deathlike convulsions are followed by a just-as-swift return to life. Then the person may recount strange, supernatural experiences, of journeys like Mohammed's, hearing the voice of God, sensing evil presences, among many others. The psychologist C. G. Jung had a boy patient with epilepsy who was terrorized by threatening, deathlike figures.

The epileptic experience of leaving the body and looking down on oneself is very much like the near-death experiences reported widely today. As both an internal experience and an observed phenomenon, a seizure resembles death, the ultimate dissolution of the known order. That rebirth quickly follows only adds to its strangeness.

A seizure's pattern of death and rebirth has yielded the deepest insights for me. The experience is one of a symbolic death and rebirth of the kind the psychologist/anthropologist Richard Katz describes vividly:

> During the experience of psychological death you give up who you are, what you are accustomed to. And in the process of giving up your identity, you can enter the state of transcendance. The conviction that you will be reborn encourages you to enter this state. You can accept the fear, it is no longer immobilizing—as when you fear that you will become nothing or that you can't come back again to yourself. . . . The basic process is being able to accept the unknown, to willingly go into fundamental mysteries.[2]

These words have illuminated for me the experience of the dissolution of order in that massive seizure now years ago.

When I relax and dispel the growing terror with deep, slow breaths, it is an act in accepting the fear, the unknown. In my case no great transcendent experiences have followed, but being able to accept fear, to meet the unknown, to risk the momentary loss of self is experience enough.

Persons who do have strange psychic or religious experiences face a particular dilemma. These episodes may have real value in themselves, both to the person and possibly to society, and I am puzzled and perplexed about the question of taking medications or using any methods that eliminate them. The nineteenth-century neurologist Hughlings Jackson called these experiences "portals," doorways to "the beyond or the unknown." We need to remember that St. Paul's hearing the voice of God on the road to Damascus may have been a seizure. Dostoyevski found his experience of religious ecstasy worth the price of epilepsy. The intuitions brought to practical purposes by people like Harriet Tubman might be lost to our societal impoverishment. The special status and potential attributed to epilepsy in some other societies reminds us of the limitations of our own western view. A seizure may be more or other than an unacceptable neurophysiological event that should be eliminated.

I am convinced that anyone who experiences the strange episodes accompanying many seizure patterns should consider seriously whether he or she wishes to eliminate them as part of seizure control. I suggest that you ask yourself if these episodes enrich your life in some way. Do they contribute to your creativity? Do they strengthen your spiritual or religious life? Does the visual imagery suggest new possibilities for your painting or drawing? Do the preliminary events bring unusual insights? You may not wish to lose these experiences. In his remarkable book, The Man Who Mistook His Wife for a Hat, the neurologist Oliver Sacks writes, "There are epilepsies which are exciting . . . . but there are other epilepsies which bring peace and well-being. A wellness can be genuine even if caused by an illness. And such a paradoxical wellness may even confer a lasting benefit."[3]

You will need to balance these experiences against the requirements of a more or less normal life. Are your seizures either infrequent enough or mild enough to be endurable? Is it possible to lead a reasonably normal life without taking the medication necessary for control? Can you maintain a self-care regimen based on the material in this book that will give you sufficient control so that family, work, friendships, and driving are not jeopardized? No one can answer these questions for another person.

In looking back over the decades of my own experience with epilepsy I come to the conclusion that I would approach it much differently now than I did. As soon as it was diagnosed, I would begin to learn about it, reading everything available, instead of fearing to be seen leaving the public library with a book branded "epilepsy" on its cover. Once I had gone for two years seizure-free on anticonvulsant medication, I would ease off the drugs, taking a year or more to do it. By this means my body would be relieved of the burden of their toxicity, and my spirit would be lifted from the chronic fatigue and depression the phenobarbital and Dilantin exacerbated. Today a neurologist would advise and help with such a change. Meanwhile I would make the changes in life-style, diet, and stress release that have served me well since I inadvertently stumbled upon them. A neurologist like Joel Reiter and an epilepsy counselor like Donna Andrews, or a seizures workshop course, would give me every assistance in making these changes.

Whenever a seizure seemed to threaten, I would use the calming thoughts and deep relaxing breaths that have succeeded for me as a way to arrest naturally a seizure's onset. Afterward I would restrict my driving until I was sure my equilibrium had returned. Then I would address the images and feelings of the aura with a psychotherapist experienced with dreams, images, and symbols. The images would then take on meaning and be available, an "open book" like the one that appeared on my coffee table as that massive seizure began years ago. In short, I would live a vastly improved quality of life that would have spilled over into the lives of my always concerned husband and my sons as they grew and developed.

That is what I would have done, I am convinced, if I had known then what I know now about epilepsy. My life did not go that way but I am grateful that I eventually learned what I have learned, for it has helped me immeasurably.

And I am grateful for more than that. To anyone interested in literature, epilepsy is the richest possible opportunity. Through it and because of it I have read some of the great literature of the world that I was not acquainted with: the writings of Hippocrates and Galen, of Paracelsus and St. Teresa of Ávila, of the great neurologists of the last two centuries, Hughlings Jackson and William Gowers, Jean Charcot, Wilder Penfield, and Oliver Sacks, of the marvelous historians of medicine, Owsei Temkin and Ludwig Edelstein, with their footnotes in Latin and Greek. Of equal value was the opportunity to read again with new eyes and insight the great literature of epilepsy: *Silas Marner,* "Julius Caesar," Dostoyevski, the contemporary novel *The Episode,* and the play, " 'night, Mother," to bring a deeper response to the film *Mean Streets.*

I am doubtful that having epilepsy has enhanced my writing or my imagination. Dostoyevski's seizures probably began in the right hemisphere, the more imaginative side, whereas the focus of mine is in the left. Nevertheless, I do hope, as Pascal did in his "Prayer to Ask of God the Proper Use of Sickness," that I have made "proper use" of it. I hope that you may find, through reading this book, new value in the epileptic experiences that occur within the context of your own life and experience.

What does the future hold for epilepsy? It will bring change, perhaps dramatic change. Research in epilepsy is ongoing, and it is continually revealing new data and modifying former conclusions. In the last weeks of preparing this book for publication, Dr. Joel Reiter and I have updated and added new material. The neurosciences are the most dynamic area of medical research today, and they will continue to be so for the foreseeable future.

Much of the research on the brain has always been done on—or with—people with epilepsy. When the Canadian neurosurgeon Wilder Penfield stimulated the different areas of the brain during surgery on patients with epilepsy and reported his findings in his book, *Epilepsy and the Func-*

tional Anatomy of the Human Brain, he was not the first researcher or the last. Epilepsy figured in the research on the separate functions of the left and right hemispheres of the brain. During surgery for intractable seizures the corpus collosum, the bridge between the hemispheres, was severed. Such research with its dramatic insights will continue. New findings on how the brain functions will influence the diagnosis and treatment of epilepsy.

Most recently, new interpretations of electroencephalograms have emerged. When the brain's electrical activity is seen in a new light, views of epilepsy and its treatment may be altered. New discoveries in the brain's biochemistry will also make changes. More effective and less toxic medications may result, and dietary control of seizures is entirely possible. Investigation continues in psychoneuroimmunology, the ways in which the mind, our attitudes and convictions, affect our diseases and disorders, even the course and speed of the aging process. More will be learned about the ways in which we bring conscious purpose to bear on brain mechanism. These new insights will be applied to the treatment of epilepsy, as will new information from magnetic resonance imaging and PET scans (Positron Emission Tomography, which pictures blood flow to parts of the brain as they are being used) as well as even newer high-tech means of diagnosis.

Besides the changes that will come through scientific research, the culture in which we live will change. Perhaps a new and higher regard for epilepsy will emerge. It may well be seen not as a threatening event to be controlled or eliminated but as an indication of the neurological basis for potentially superlative artistic achievement and highly creative activity in many spheres.

It is my hope that this book will contribute to a new view of epilepsy's value.

ADDENDUM I

Special Concerns for Women with Epilepsy

In the first epilepsy support group that I joined in the early 1980s, a woman described her seizures to us. They struck just before her period began, and her doctor had told her it was all psychological and she should see a psychiatrist. She was upset and confused, and understandably so. Today the phenomenon of seizures at menstruation is recognized in medicine and is dignified with a name, catamenial epilepsy.

For years women's health, outside of childbearing, was slighted by the medical establishment. Only recently have women's health issues been recognized as distinct from men's. Research is finally being conducted on the special medical concerns of women.

Gender does affect the course of epilepsy, beginning at birth and continuing into old age.

From infancy through adulthood, girls and boys go through similar stages of development, but not necessarily at the same age. Pubescence is the most obvious example, although not the only one. In spite of the general conviction that puberty increases the risk of epilepsy, among most researchers today, writes Martha Morrell, M.D., of Stanford University, "there is general agreement that seizure frequency is not substantially altered at puberty"[1] in either sex. Some "transient worsening" may occur, and certain seizure types may be more or less likely to appear, but contemporary research does not support the kind of parental

246

fear I have heard so often expressed, that seizures will get worse once a child becomes pubescent.

Women are less vulnerable to epilepsy than men, and most types of seizures afflict more males than females, with some exceptions. Partial and complex partial seizures, childhood absence, and photosensitive seizures are more common among women. The seizures associated with Rett syndrome and Aicardi syndrome occur exclusively in females. Both syndromes indicate severely delayed development. "When prolonged lateralized febrile seizures occur in early life, girls seem more vulnerable to severe effects than boys."[2] The threat that infant febrile seizures will become generalized seizures lasts through the first year of life for girls but throughout childhood for boys. Seizures from head injury are much less common among girls.

In recent years medical attention and research have focused on hormones and their complexities throughout life for both men and women. "Sex hormones influence brain function as early as day 40 of gestation," writes Martha Morrell, M.D.,[3] but they become primary factors after puberty. When the female hormone estrogen is high, as it is just before menstruation, seizure thresholds lower. Progesterone raises seizure thresholds by diminishing cortical excitability. At the time of menstruation the balance between estrogen and progesterone changes; the change in balance of the two hormones is believed to account for catamenial seizures.

Menstrual difficulties, infertility, and other reproductive endocrine abnormalities are much more common among women with epilepsy than among the general female population. Some researchers see epilepsy itself as causal. Certain types of seizures—temporal lobe epilepsy with a left hemisphere focus, for instance—seem to increase susceptibility. Other researchers put the blame on anticonvulsant medications, valproate especially. The intricate interactions of hormones, seizure type, and anticonvulsant medication make for further complications in an already complicated condition.

These volatile aspects carry over into issues around

pregnancy. First of all, barrier methods of contraception are recommended for most women with epilepsy since antiepileptic drugs can nullify the protective action of the pill. With barrier methods like a diaphragm or condom or both, accidental pregnancy is less likely to occur. Since the first three months are a period of critical development for the fetus, that's when the fetus is most vulnerable to malformations from epileptic medication. Therefore, the damage to the infant could be done before a woman knows she is pregnant. Joel Reiter discusses the pros and cons of "'Antiepileptic Medication During Pregnancy" in chapter 5, and I urge every woman who is considering pregnancy to read those pages. In addition, any woman who might have a child through a planned or accidental pregnancy should take a multiple vitamin supplement with folic acid, for it tends to protect against birth defects.[4]

The Portland, Oregon, neurologist Marc Yerby, M.D., has emerged as a leading authority on pregnancy and epilepsy. He recommends the following:[5]

1. Prenatal care including visits to a neurologist during pregnancy.
2. Good nutrition and a 25–30 pound weight gain (chapter 16).
3. No smoking, no caffeine, no alcohol, no hard drugs (chapter 18).
4. Reduce stress and get plenty of rest. Exercise by walking (chapters 13 and 14).
5. Avoid pesticides, oven cleaner, and other strong chemicals (chapter 19).

(See chapters following individual guidelines for help in planning a personal program.)

In Dr. Yerby's opinion, a woman should continue with her medication because the risk of birth defects is not great and less than the possible harm from a seizure.

At menopause, women face another period of hormonal volatility—estrogen levels drop in relation to progesterone. Consequently, seizure activity may decline. For some women whose bones lose density (osteoporosis) after menopause, hormone (estrogen) replacement therapy is often recommended. With this therapy menstruation resumes, as may seizures. Women with epilepsy must look at this choice in the context of their total health picture. I know of no research that addresses this issue. Supplemental calcium and moderate exercise with some easy weight lifting make up an effective substitute therapy, and they are often recommended in addition to estrogen replacement.

In the past some women with epilepsy have been judged to have below normal sexual urges. Today this condition is often blamed on anticonvulsant medication, but a long history of seizures, especially complex partial seizures, a temporal lobe focus, and menstrual abnormalities all have an effect in lowering the sex drive. In my view hyposexuality is only a problem if your partner complains. In that case, you will find some help in chapter 15.

As reports of wife battering rise, another sad fact emerges. The trauma sustained during beatings is blamed by a number of women for causing epileptic seizures. Anyone who finds herself or her children subject to physical or sexual abuse should take immediate measures to ensure her safety and her children's. Women's shelters can provide temporary housing and long-term assistance.

Childhood sexual abuse is also seen by more researchers as a factor in psychogenic seizures (pseudoseizures). The British team of Tim Betts and Sarah Boden concludes that a seizure with unconsciousness is a way to block the memory of abuse, whereas an abreactive seizure suggests a kind of acting out of the abuse.[6]

Cardiovascular disease is the principal cause of new epilepsy cases among older people. Until recently women's heart problems did not receive the attention given to men's. Heart disease tends to occur later in life for women. Today, as women carry more of the economic burden, the medical attitude toward female heart disease has changed considerably. There are many concerns for older women with epilepsy. For further discussion of seizures among older women, see Addendum II: Special Concerns for Older People with Epilepsy.

If you want to read more about women's special concerns, the best book I know of is *Women and Epilepsy* (1991), edited by M. R. Trimble, an eminent British epileptologist. Although not widely available, it can be ordered from John Wiley and Sons, New York, New York. The ISBN number is 0-471-92998-0.

ADDENDUM II

Special Concerns for Older People with Epilepsy

"And now I'm an epileptic!" the man of seventy exclaimed to me. "What am I going to do?"

"Think of yourself as a person with seizures, for starters," I said, "not as an epileptic."

This older man's shock and horror at his newly diagnosed condition are common reactions to epilepsy at any age. However, the aging process is complex and difficult at best; suddenly having to cope with seizures compounds the problems.

Not long ago the medical community believed that epilepsy rarely set in after the age of fifty or so. As the elderly population has increased and has had more access to doctors because of Medicare, the health of older people has come under greater surveillance. It is also the subject of more research than ever before. The incidence of new cases of epilepsy in people over fifty has reached some 30,000 a year, about equal to the incidence in early childhood. The causes, however, are quite different.

"The majority of [these] new onset seizures are secondary to cardiovascular disease," Dr. Joel Reiter writes, "either thrombosis or cardiac embolism. Some [are caused] by strokes. Many are silent strokes." A transient ischemic attack (TIA) will momentarily reduce the amount of oxygen flowing to the brain and may leave seizures in its wake. When an embolism, a blood clot, reaches the brain through arterial pathways, the subsequent stroke may cause seizures. It did so in the case of the older man quoted above. What's more, the neurological damage of the initial attack can be worsened by persistent seizures.

A developing brain tumor is another cause, although tumors are much less common among people over seventy than among younger folks.

Some 50 to 70 percent of the cases of epilepsy among older people can be attributed to known causes. The remainder are of unknown origin. When seizures occur because of other diseases and conditions, they are considered to be "secondary epilepsy," that is, a consequence of that other disease.[1]

Older people's cases can be complicated by other conditions. Late-onset diabetes may be undiagnosed. The aging body may no longer be able to tolerate long-term abuse of alcohol or habitual poor nutrition. Older people average— average!—five prescription drugs a day, and the interaction of one drug with another can cause seizures. Declining exercise and loss of muscle tone and the general low resistance characteristic of aging may make the person more vulnerable and lower his or her seizure threshold.

Seizures from psychological causes are rare after sixty. Nonetheless, they do occur and for the same reasons as those that affect younger people: deep-running emotional tensions, unresolved issues, and a childhood history of physical and sexual abuse.

Recurring bouts of memory loss may be of epileptic origin and are frequent enough to have acquired a name, "epileptic amnesiac attacks." They are not necessarily linked to pervasive mental deterioration. The possibility of other causes such as advanced Alzheimer's disease can be confirmed or ruled out diagnostically.

Seizures may appear after serious falls and accidents. Unsteadiness on their feet and vision impairment make the elderly more susceptible to such accidents.

If all this sounds like bad news, the mortality statistics are only somewhat more cheering. In and of itself epilepsy is rarely the primary cause of death. But when it occurs as a complicating factor along with brain tumor or cardiovascular disease, the death rate is much higher than it is among persons who have those conditions but no seizures.[2]

These causes and complications are serious. When seizures occur, the older person must seek medical advice promptly or be helped to do so. A thorough neurological workup with EEG, CT-scan, and perhaps an MRI (magnetic resonance imaging), as well as a thorough cardiological workup will identify some causes. Brain tumor surgery for older people has a record of success. Prompt treatment increases the chances of getting seizures under control and reducing them as a complicating factor.

What treatment regimens are recommended? Dr. Joel Reiter tells me that he finds quite low dosages of anticonvulsants effective for older people, and the research confirms this. Phenytoin (Dilantin) is the drug of choice, and single-drug therapy is preferred. A review of drug-drug interactions may help the person improve in health and functioning by eliminating those drugs that oppose or negate essential medications.

Of course, it is also important to detect and treat any other physical problems that may be present, such as diabetes, alcoholism, hypothyroidism, or hyperglycemia (high blood sugar).[3] When good seizure control is achieved, as is often the case, a slow reduction of anticonvulsant may be possible.

Cardiovascular problems can be detected during a thorough medical examination, and they, too, can be treated successfully. In addition, the relaxation methods presented in chapters 13, 14, and 15 will prove helpful. Cardiological research studies show that meditation and deep relaxation lower blood pressure and relieve hypertension and stress. There has been no research that I know of on the effectiveness of these methods specifically for older people whose heart problems have brought on seizures. But the success of these methods with a younger population suggests that they would succeed. They are certainly worth a try. All of the self-care methods for prevention and intervention presented in this book will be helpful at any age.

Seizures & Seniors, a pamphlet put out by the Epilepsy Foundation of America, summarizes the basic information on epilepsy and older people. It has some good suggestions for making life safer. The pamphlet is available through the EFA. For the address see page 136.

As I grow older, I wonder from time to time if my seizures will break through again. (I have had no seizures in ten years.) If they should, I shall follow my own advice and take these six steps:

1. See my doctor immediately and have thorough cardiological and neurological workups.
2. Review my life-style, drug intake, and nutrition.
3. Try to detect an aura and create a behavioral intervention.
4. Practice methods for stress reduction and greater relaxation.
5. If my neurologist prescribes it, take a low dosage of a single anticonvulsant until seizures are controlled.

My own preference would be to taper off medication, if possible, but Joel Reiter tells me that most older people, especially those with grand mal (tonic-clonic) seizures, will need antiepileptic medication for the remainder of their lives.

When epilepsy occurs among the elderly, causes may be somewhat different than in a younger group, but they are addressed in much the same ways with medication, possible surgery, changes of life-style, and control or elimination of complicating factors. In addition, Joel Reiter and I are convinced that all the health-enhancing self-care programs laid out in this book will help older people as much as they help younger ones.

NOTES

CHAPTER 1

1. Cousins, Norman, "The Mysterious Placebo: How Mind Helps Medicine Work," *Saturday Review*, October 1, 1977, p. 16.

2. Efron, Robert, "The Conditioned Inhibition of Uncinate Fits," *Brain* 1957, pp. 251–261.

3. Ibid., p. 251.

4. Green, Elmer, and Alyce Green, *Beyond Biofeedback*. Delacorte, New York, 1977, pp. 103–106.

5. Valeo, Tom, "A Glimpse of How Mind Produces Art," *Boston Globe*, January 16, 1989, p. 48.

CHAPTER 2

1. Katz, Richard, lecture, Harvard University, November 1987.

2. Shem, Samuel, (pseud.) "Journeyings in the Land of the 'Seventh Sense'," *Boston Globe*, December 29, 1985, p. A13.

3. Kleinman, Arthur, *Patients and Healers in the Context of Culture*. University of California Press, Berkeley, 1980.

4. Benson, Herbert, and William Proctor, *Your Maximum Mind*. Times Books, New York, 1987.

5. Callaghan, Noel, Andrew Garrett, and Timothy Goggin, "Withdrawal of anticonvulsant drugs in patients free of seizures for two years," *New England Journal of Medicine*, April 14, 1988, p. 942.

6. Shinnar, Shlomo, Eileen P. G. Vining, E. David Mellits, Bernard J. D'Souza, Kenton Holden, Rosemary A. Baumgardnes, and John G. Freeman, "Discontinuing Antiepileptic Medications in Children with Epilepsy After Two Years Without Seizures," *New England Journal of Medicine*, October 17, 1985, pp. 976–980.

7. LaPlante, Eve, "Medicine: The Riddle of TLE," *Atlantic*, October 1988, p. 34.

8. Valeo, op. cit.

9. Sacks, Oliver, *The Man Who Mistook His Wife for a Hat*. Summit Books, New York, 1985, p. 139.

10. Reiter, Joel, Donna Andrews, and Charlotte Janis, *Taking Control of Your Epilepsy*. Andrews/Reiter Epilepsy Research Program, Inc., Santa Rosa, Calif., 1987.

CHAPTER 3
1. Lennox, W. and M. Lennox, *Epilepsy and Related Disorders*, Little, Brown and Co., Boston, 1960, p. 53.
2. Tempkin, Oswei, *The Falling Sickness*, 2nd ed., The Johns Hopkins Press, Baltimore, 1971.
3. Adams, F., *The Extant Works of Aretaeus, the Cappadocian*, reprint of 1856 edition, Wertheimer and Co., London, 1972, p. 245.
4. Laidlaw, J., and A. Richens, *A Textbook of Epilepsy*, Churchill Livingstone, London, 1982, p. 97.

CHAPTER 4
1. Laidlaw, J., and A. Richens, *A Textbook of Epilepsy*, Churchill Livingstone, London, p. 128.
2. Engel, Jerome, *Seizures and Epilepsy*, F. A. Davis Co., Philadelphia, 1989.

Surgical treatment of epilepsy:

3. Spencer, Susan, "Surgical options for uncontrolled epilepsy," *Neurological Clinics* 4 (3): 669–695, 1986.

CHAPTER 5
1. Joynt, R., editor, *Clinical Neurology*, revised ed., volume 3, J. B. Lippincott, Co., Philadelphia, 1988, p. 58.
2. Lennox, W. and M. Lennox, *Epilepsy and Related Disorders*, Little, Brown and Co., Boston, 1960, p. 821.
3. Tempkin, Oswei, *The Falling Sickness*, 2nd ed., The Johns Hopkins Press, Baltimore, 1971.
4. Lyons, K. L., R. V. Lacro, et al., "Pattern of Malformations in the Children of Women Treated with Carbamazepine During Pregnancy," *New England Journal of Medicine* 320: 1661–1666, 1989.
5. Jones, Kenneth Lyons, personal communication, June 1989.

CHAPTER 6
1. LeBaron, Gaye, "A long walk to the podium," *The Press Democrat*, Santa Rosa, California, May 31, 1989, p. A2.
2. Lennox, W., and M. Lennox, *Epilepsy and Related Disorders*, Little, Brown and Co., Boston, 1960, p. 1066.
3. Eliot, R., "Coronary artery disease: biobehavioral factors," *Circulation* II (76), no. 1 (supplement I), pp. I–111, July, 1987.
4. Lown, B., "Sudden cardiac death: Biobehavioral perspective," *Circulation* II (76), no. 1 (supplement I), pp. I–194, July, 1987.
5. Friedman, M., R. H. Rosenman, V. Carroll, "Changes in the serum cholesterol and blood clotting time in men subjected to cyclic variation of occupational stress," *Circulation* 17, 1958, p. 852.
6. Ornish, D., *Abstracts of the Society of Behavioral Medicine 10th Anniversary Meeting 1989*, and personal communication with Dr. Michael Samuels.

7. Grant, I., and L. Temoshok, et al., *Abstracts of the Society of Behavioral Medicine 10th Anniversary Meeting,* 1989.

8. Lynch, J., *The Language of the Heart,* Basic Books, Inc., New York, 1985, p. 261. (Dr. Lynch quotes from Dr. Cannon's seminal work, *Bodily Changes in Pain, Hunger, Fear and Rage: An Account of Recent Researches into the Function of Emotional Excitement,* Appleton, New York, 1929.)

CHAPTER 7

1. Penfield, Wilder, and Herbert Jasper, *Epilepsy and the Functional Anatomy of the Human Brain,* Little, Brown and Co., Boston, 1954, p. 564.

2. Simonton, Carl, and Stephanie Simonton, *Getting Well Again,* J. P. Tarcher, Los Angeles, 1978.

3. Benson, Herbert, and Miriam Z. Klipper, *The Relaxation Response,* Avon, New York, 1976.

4. Sacks, op. cit., p. 4.

5. Mauriac, François (ed.), *The Living Thoughts of Pascal,* Cassell and Co., Ltd., London, 1941. pp. 28–39.

6. Ibid., p. 38.

7. Penfield, op. cit., p. 564.

8. Mendez, M. F., J. L. Cummings, and D. Frank Benson, "Depression in Epilepsy," *Archives of Neurology,* 43:766–770, August 1986.

9. Gross, Meir, "Incestuous Rape," *Journal of the American Orthopsychiatric Association,* pp. 704–708, 1979.

10. Ibid., p. 708.

11. Cousins, Norman, *Christian Science Monitor,* November 13, 1987.

12. Sacks, Oliver, *Migraine.* University of California Press, Berkeley, 1985.

CHAPTER 8

1. Alajouanine, F., "Dostoyevski's Epilepsy," *Brain* 86:214–218, June 1963.

2. Sacks, op. cit., p. 139.

3. Jung, Carl G., *Collected Works,* Princeton University Press, Princeton, New Jersey: vol. 8, p. 582.

4. Bear, David, lecture, conference on "Art and the Brain," Art Institute of Chicago, 1988.

5. Ezekiel 26:1, 42:1–19, 43:13–17.

6. Teresa of Avila, *The Interior Castle,* The Paulist Press, New Jersey, 1979 (originally 1577), p. 131.

7. Ibid., p. 133.

8. James, William, *The Varieties of Religious Experience,* Modern Library, New York, 1936 (originally 1902), p. 8.

9. Schoern, Max, *The Psychology of Music,* American Biography Service, Inc., 1940, Reprint Services Corp., Irvine, CA, p. 105.

10. Kanner, Otto, "The Names of the Falling Sickness," *Human Biology,* vol. 2. Johns Hopkins Press, Baltimore, 1930, p. 116.

11. James, William, op. cit., p. 15.

12. Ibid., p. 15.

13. Grof, Stanislav, and Christina Grof, "Forms of Spiritual Emergency," *Spiritual Emergency Network Newsletter*, California Institute of Transpersonal Psychology, Menlo Park, 1985.

CHAPTER 9

1. Temkin, Oswei, *The Falling Sickness*, The Johns Hopkins Press, Baltimore, 1971 (originally 1945), p. 14.

2. Hippocrates, "On the Sacred Disease," *Hippocrates and Galen*, The Great Books, vol. 10, Encyclopaedia Britannica, Chicago, p. 154.

3. Ibid., p. 155.

4. Jung, C. G., *Mandala Symbolism*. Princeton University Press, Princeton, N.J., 1972, pp. 3–4.

5. Mark 9:14 ff.

6. Easterbrook, Gregg, "The Business of Politics," *Atlantic*, October 1986, p. 36.

7. "From Medical Directions Written for Governor Winthrop of Massachusetts by Dr. Stafford of London, 1643," *Harvard Medical Alumni Bulletin*, Summer 1986, p. 53.

8. Willis, Sir Thomas, *The Anatomy of the Brain and Nerves*, McGill University Press, Montreal, Quebec, Canada, 1966 (originally 1664).

9. Temkin, op. cit., p. 299.

10. Bear, David, lecture on "Art and the Brain," Chicago, 1988.

11. Gelfand, Michael, "The African's Concept of Causes and Treatment of Epilepsy and Convulsions," *South Africa Medical Journal*, April 27, 1974, pp. 879–881.

12. Watson, Lyall, *Lightning Bird*, Dutton, New York, 1982, p. 88.

13. Eliade, Mircea, *Shamanism*, Princeton University Press, Princeton, N.J., 1964.

14. Kleinman, op. cit., p. 311 ff.

CHAPTER 10

1. Cohen, Morton N., ed., *The Selected Letters of Lewis Carroll*. Pantheon Books, New York, 1982, p. 205.

CHAPTER 11

1. Noakes, Vivian, *Edward Lear*, Houghton Mifflin Co., Boston, 1969, p. 112.

2. Hippocrates, op. cit., p. 156.

CHAPTER 12

1. Penfield, Wilder, *The Mystery of the Mind*, Princeton University Press, Princeton, N.J., 1975, p. 46.

CHAPTER 13

1. Carroll, Lewis, op. cit., p. 205.

2. Snyder, Mariah, "Stressor Inventory for Persons with Epilepsy," *Journal of Neuroscience Nursing* 18(2):71–73, April 1986.

CHAPTER 14

1. Noakes, op. cit., p. 78.
2. Ibid., p. 110.
3. Snyder, Mariah, "Effect of Relaxation on Psychosocial Functioning in Persons with Epilepsy," *Journal of Neurosurgical Nursing* 15(4):250–254, August 1983.
4. Ibid., p. 251.
5. Dahl, J., L. Melin, L. Lund, "Effects of a Contingent Relaxation Treatment Program on Adults with Refractory Epilepsy Seizures," *Epilepsia*, 28:125–132, 1987.
6. Legion, Vivian, personal correspondence with Joel Reiter, March 5, 1990.
7. Borysenko, Joan, instruction sheet, Mind/Body Clinic, New England Deaconess Hospital–Harvard Medical School Department of Behavioral Medicine, Boston.
8. Ibid., an adaptation.

CHAPTER 15

1. Borysenko, Joan, *Minding the Body, Mending the Mind*, Addison-Wesley, Burlington, Mass., 1987, p. 61.
2. Benson, Herbert, and William Proctor, *Beyond the Relaxation Response*, Times Books, New York, 1984, p. 99.

CHAPTER 16

1. Brody, Jane, *Jane Brody's the New York Times Guide to Personal Health*, Times Books, New York, 1982, pp. xiii, xvii.
2. Dreher, Henry, *Your Defense Against Cancer*, Harper & Row, New York, 1989, pp. 147–171.
3. Albertson, T. E., R. M. Joy, and L. G. Stark, "Caffeine Modification of Kindled Amygdaloid Seizures," *Pharmacology, Biochemistry, and Behavior*, Pergamon Journals, Elmsford, N.Y. vol. 19, 1983, pp. 339–343.
4. White, James C., letter, *The New England Journal of Medicine*, vol. 312 (4), 1985, p. 246.

CHAPTER 17

1. Hippocrates, op. cit., p. 157.
2. Pfeiffer, Carl C., *Nutritional Control of Seizures*, Princeton Brain Bio Center, Skillman, N.J.
3. McCann, Kevin, Donald P. Cain, and Diana J. Philbrick, "Facilitation of Kindled Seizures in Rats Fed Choline-Supplemented Diets," *Canadian Journal of Neurological Sciences*, vol. 10 (1), February 1983, pp. 47–49.
4. *The Graedons' People's Pharmacy Guide to Nutrient and Drug Reactions*, 1985. King Features, 235 E. 45th St., New York, N.Y. 10017.
5. Current research on the role of vitamin E in treating epilepsy from Children's Hospital, Oakland, California; cited by Dr. K. Laxer at the February, 1990 meeting of the San Francisco Neurological Society.

CHAPTER 18
1. Hulsker, Jan., ed. *Van Gogh's 'Diary'*, William Morrow and Co., New York, 1971, p. 103.
2. *National Spokesman*, Epilepsy Foundation of America newsletter, "Alcohol and Epilepsy," October 1988, p. 10.
3. Ibid., p. 11.
4. *Tufts University Diet and Nutrition Letter*, vol. 4, no. 1, March 1986. Tufts University Diet and Nutrition Letter, 53 Park Place, 8th floor, New York, New York 10007.
5. Dreher, Henry, op. cit., p. 84.
6. Tye, Larry, "Small Dose Can Be Fatal, Study Says," *Boston Globe*, September 25, 1986, p. 1.
7. Ibid.

CHAPTER 19
1. Goetz, Christopher G., Harold L. Klawans, and Maynard M. Cohen, "Neurotoxic Agents," *Clinical Neurology*, vol. 2, Harper & Row, Philadelphia, 1987, p. 31.
2. Ibid, pp. 5–9.
3. Ibid., p. 3
4. Ibid., p. 9.
5. Ibid., pp. 19–20.
6. "The Mind," PBS TV, 1988.
7. Goetz et al., op. cit., p. 1.
8. Gilbert, Mary E., "Formamidine Pesticides Enhance Susceptibility to Kindled Seizures in Amygdala and Hippocampus of the Rat," *Neurotoxicology and Teratology*, vol. 10, Pergamon Press, Elmsford, N.Y., 1988, p. 221.
9. Joy, Robert M., "The Effects of Neurotoxicants on Kindling and Kindled Seizures," *Fundamental and Applied Toxicology* 5:59, 1985.
10. Gilbert, M. E., C. M. Mack, and K. M. Crofton, "Pyrethroids and Enhanced Inhibition in the Hippocampus of the Rat," *Brain Research* 477:314–321, Elsevier, 1989.
11. Joy, op. cit., p. 43.
12. Gilbert, Mary E., personal correspondence, May 24, 1989.

CHAPTER 20
1. Efron, op. cit., p. 251.
2. Penfield, op. cit., p. 39.
3. Efron, op. cit., p. 261.
4. Penfield, op. cit., p. 39.
5. Efron, op. cit., p. 253.
6. Ibid., p. 260.
7. Penfield, op. cit., p. 39.
8. Pritchard, Paul B., III, Valerie L. Holmstrom, and Joseph Giacinto, "Self-Abatement of Complex Partial Seizures," *Annals of Neurology* 18:265–267, 1985.
9. Penfield, op. cit., p. 39.
10. Pritchard, op. cit., p. 266.

11. Ibid., p. 266.

12. Ibid., p. 266.

13. Penry, Kiffin, "The Behavioral Aspects of Seizures," American Psychiatric Association Annual Meeting, 1988.

14. Feldman, Robert G., and N. N. Paul, "Identity of Emotional Triggers in Epilepsy," *Journal of Nervous and Mental Disease* 162 (5):345–353, May 1976.

15. Penfield, op. cit., p. 39.

CHAPTER 21

1. Zlutnick, Steven, William J. Mayville, and Scott Moffat, "Modification of Seizure Disorders: The Interruption of Behavioral Chains," *Annual Review of Behavior Therapy (Journal of Applied Behavior Analysis)* 8:1–12, 476, 1975.

2. Forster, F. M., "Conditional Reflex Therapy in Epilepsy," *Georgetown Medical Bulletin*, vol. 21, 1967; Flannery, R. B., and J. R. Cautela, "Seizures: Controlling the Uncontrollable," *Journal of Rehabilitation*, vol. 39, 1973; Feldman, R. G., and N. N. Paul, op. cit.; Mostofsky, David, and Barbara Balaschak, op. cit.; Fenwick, Peter, "Precipitation and Inhibition of Seizures," *Epilepsy and Psychiatry*. Reynolds and Trimble, editors, Edinburgh, Scotland: Churchill Livingstone, 1981; Chadwick, David, and E. H. Reynolds, "When do epileptic patients need treatment?" *British Medical Journal*, vol. 290, 1985; and Dahl, JoAnne, L. Melin, and P. Lessner, "Effects of a Behavioral Intervention on Epileptic Seizures Behavior and Paroxysmal Activity," *Epilepsia* 29:2, 1988.

3. Dahl, JoAnne, *Epilepsy; A Behavior Medicine Approach*, Hofgrefe and Huber, Seattle, 1992.

4. Cautela, Joseph R., "The Self-Control Triad," *Behavior Modification* 7(3):299–315, 1983.

5. Dahl, JoAnne, Lo Brorson, Lennart Melin, "Effects of a Broad-Spectrum Behavioral Medicine Treatment Program: An 8-Year Follow-up," *Epilepsia* 33(1):98–102, 1992.

6. Zlutnick et al., op. cit.

7. Cautela, op. cit.

CHAPTER 22

1. Basmajian, J., *Biofeedback Principles and Practice for Clinicians*, 2nd ed., J. V. Basmajian, ed., Williams & Wilkins, Baltimore, 1983, p. 1.

2. Whitman, Steven, et. al., *Progressive Relaxation for Seizure Reduction*, publication of the Center for Urban Affairs and Policy Research, Northwestern University, Evanston, Ill., 1989.

3. Lynch, J., *The Language of the Heart*, Basic Books, Inc., New York, 1985, p. 92.

4. Basmajian, J., op. cit., p. 1.

CHAPTER 23

1. Pelletier, Kenneth B., *Mind as Healer, Mind as Slayer*, Dell Publishing Co., New York, 1977, p. 320.

2. Jaffe, Dennis, *Healing from Within*, Alfred Knopf, New York, 1980. p. 208.

CHAPTER 24

1. Pollak, Richard, "The Epilepsy Defense," *Atlantic*, May 1984, p. 20.

2. *Driving and Epilepsy*, Legal Advocacy Department, Epilepsy Foundation of America, 1986.

3. Guthrie, Dorothea, "Living with Epilepsy," *Family Safety*, National Safety Council, Chicago, Summer 1977, p. 20 ff.

4. Riesner, Helen, *Children with Epilepsy*, Woodbine House, Kensington, Md., 1987.

5. Epilepsy Foundation of America, Training and Placement Service Project, "TAPS' historical prospective."

6. Hulsker, Jan, ed., op. cit., p. 120.

7. Pollak, op, cit., pp. 20–28.

8. Levin, Ronald, Sherrie Banks, and Beverly Berg, "Psychosocial Dimensions of Epilepsy," *Epilepsia* 29 (6):805–816, 1988.

9. Pollak, op. cit., p. 28.

10. Pollak, Richard, *The Episode*, New American Library, New York, 1987.

11. Eliot, George, *Silas Marner*, New American Library, New York, 1987.

12. Pollak, Richard, "A Bitter Pill for Epileptics," *New York Times*, September 3, 1987.

CHAPTER 25

1. Sacks, Oliver, op. cit., p. 102.

2. Katz, Richard, "Education for Transcendence: Lessons from the !Kung Zhu/Twasi!" *Journal of Transpersonal Psychology* 2:153, 1973.

3. Sacks, op. cit., p. 102.

ADDENDUM I

1. Morrell, Martha J., "Hormones and Epilepsy Through the Lifetime," *Epilepsia* 33(Suppl. 4): S49–61, 1992.

2. Ibid.

3. Ibid.

4. Yerby, Marc, in *Women and Epilepsy*, M. R. Trimble, editor, John Wiley & Sons, New York, 1991.

5. Yerby, Marc, and Karen McCormick, *Pregnancy and Epilepsy* (pamphlet).

6. Betts, Tim, and Sarah Boden, "Pseudoseizures," in *Women and Epilepsy* (see note 4).

ADDENDUM II

1. Drury, Ivo, and Ahmad Beydoun, "Seizure Disorders of Aging," *Geriatrics* 48(5):52–58, 1993.

2. Luhdorf, K., L. K. Jensen, and A. M. Plesner, "Epilepsy in the Elderly," *Acta Neurologica Scandinavica* 76:183–190, 1987.

3. Morrell, op. cit.

INDEX

263